The Atlas of Layered Anatomy of Acupoints

Compiled by Gao Hualing

FOREIGN LANGUAGES PRESS   BEIJING

First Edition   1999

Home Page:
http://www.flp.com.cn
E-mail Addresses:
info@flp.com.cn
sales@flp.com.cn

ISBN 7-119-01753-5

Published by Foreign Languages Press
24 Baiwanzhuang Road, Beijing 100037, China

Printed by Foreign Languages Printing House
19 Chegongzhuang Xilu, Beijing 100044, China

Distributed by China International Book Trading Corporation
35 Chegongzhuang Xilu, Beijing 100044, China
P.O. Box 399, Beijing, China
Printed in the People's Republic of China

Contents

Preface

Acupuncture-moxibustion, essential components of traditional Chinese medicine, have many characteristics: a long history, uncomplicated, inexpensive, quickly effective and useful in a wide range of indications. They are becoming increasingly popular and accepted by both clinicians and the public at home and abroad. As for their benefits, I have summarized my many years of teaching experience to write this book, *The Atlas of Layered Anatomy of Acupoints*. It conforms to *Standard International Acupuncture Nomenclature*, which has been examined and approved by World Health Organization's (WHO) Scientific Group on International Acupuncture Nomenclature. The *Atlas* is based on meridians and points. It applies the anatomic method to draw in layered fashion, the location of points to show the relationship between the points and organs. The appendixes after the illustrations sum up the standard location of meridians and points, the posture of the patient, the direction, angle and depth of insertion of the needle, indications, the locations of the viscera beneath some points to which special attention should be paid, and selected points for common disorders.

This book will be a beneficial resource to teachers of acupuncture-moxibustion, medical researchers, acupuncturists, and medical students and individuals studying acupuncture-moxibustion.

This *Atlas* consists of two parts. The first includes the following: commonly used apparatuses, the posture of the patient, the anatomical landmarks on the surface of human body, the courses and commonly used points of the meridians, the methods of locating points, and the methods of inserting the needle. The second part contains layered illustrations of skin, muscles, vessels, nerves and skeleton, organs in each aspect of the head, trunk, upper and lower limbs, and the auricular surface. It provides a stereoscopic picture of the points, thereby furnishing readers with a complete survey.

Finally, I would like to express my great gratitude to all coworkers for their skilled performance. I am indebted to Professor Geng Enguang, who located the points, and Mr. Sheng Yingnong, who made the drawings in such an excellent manner. Thanks also to Song Fengjin, Huang Tao, Cui Xiaonan, Liu Zhilin and Gao Qiang, who offered help toward the publication of this book.

Part 1

Fig. 1 (1) The nomenclature, gauge and diameter of the needle apparatuses

Needle's name	acupuncture needle	acupuncture needle	acupuncture needle	acupuncture needle	acupuncture needle	Round-sharp needle	three-edged needle	uricular therapy	thumb-tack needle
Numder	26	28	30	32	34	21	12.16	34	32
Diameter mm	0.45	0.38	0.32	0.26	0.22				

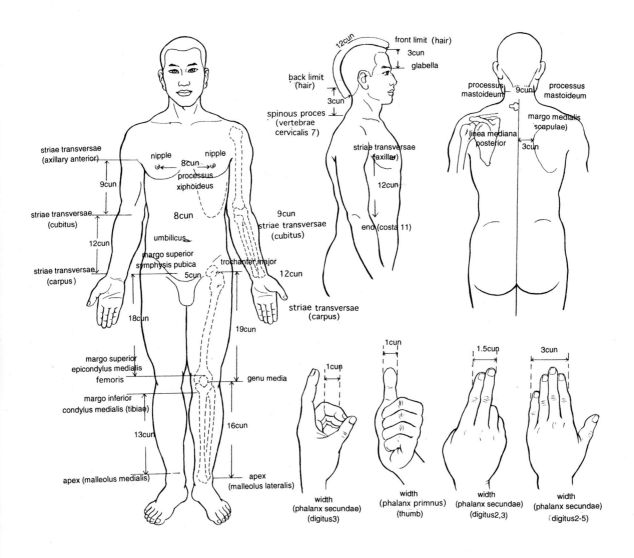

Fig. 1 (2) The cun and finger measurement on body for acupuncture-moxibustion

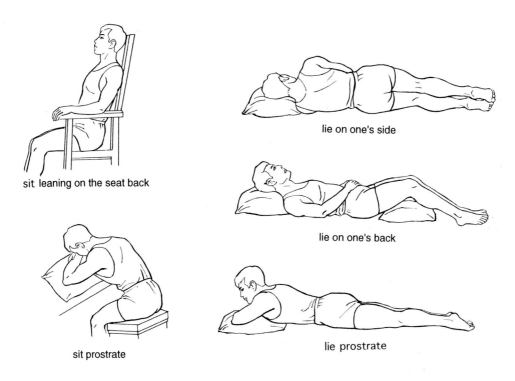

sit leaning on the seat back

lie on one's side

lie on one's back

sit prostrate

lie prostrate

Fig. 2 (1) The commonly-used postures of the patient for acupuncture-moxibustion

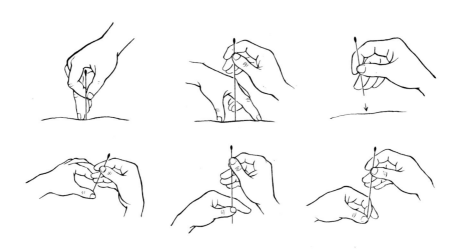

Fig. 2 (2) The directions for needle insertion

3

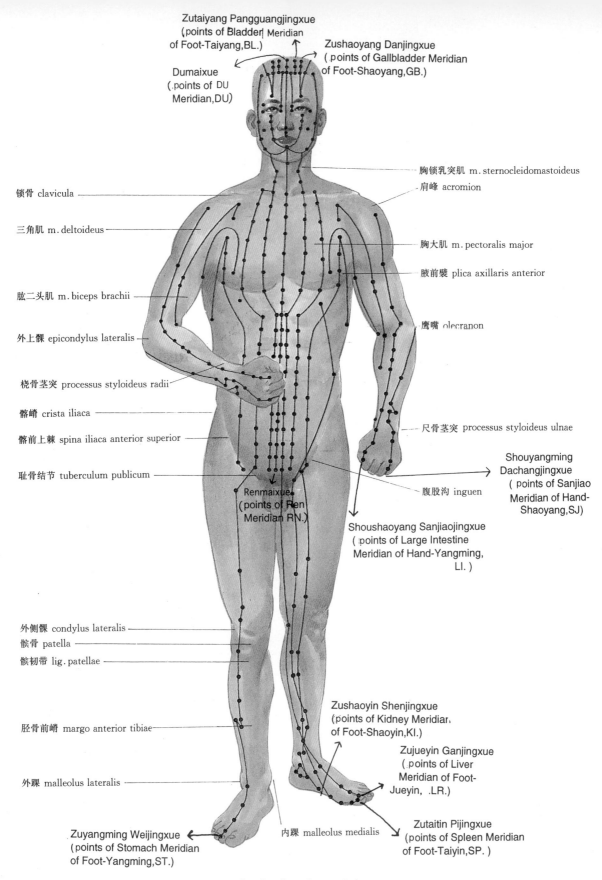

Zutaiyang Pangguangjingxue
(points of Bladder Meridian
of Foot-Taiyang,BL.)

Zushaoyang Danjingxue
(points of Gallbladder Meridian
of Foot-Shaoyang,GB.)

Dumaixue
(.points of DU
Meridian,DU)

胸锁乳突肌 m. sternocleidomastoideus

肩峰 acromion

锁骨 clavicula

三角肌 m. deltoideus

胸大肌 m. pectoralis major

腋前襞 plica axillaris anterior

肱二头肌 m. biceps brachii

鹰嘴 olecranon

外上髁 epicondylus lateralis

桡骨茎突 processus styloideus radii

髂嵴 crista iliaca

髂前上棘 spina iliaca anterior superior

尺骨茎突 processus styloideus ulnae

Shouyangming
Dachangjingxue
(points of Sanjiao
Meridian of Hand-
Shaoyang,SJ)

耻骨结节 tuberculum publicum

腹股沟 inguen

Renmaixue
(points of Ren
Meridiam RN.)

Shoushaoyang Sanjiaojingxue
(points of Large Intestine
Meridian of Hand-Yangming,
LI.)

外侧髁 condylus lateralis
髌骨 patella
髌韧带 lig. patellae

Zushaoyin Shenjingxue
(points of Kidney Meridian
of Foot-Shaoyin,KI.)

Zujueyin Ganjingxue
(.points of Liver
Meridian of Foot-
Jueyin, .LR.)

胫骨前嵴 margo anterior tibiae

外踝 malleolus lateralis

Zutaitin Pijingxue
(points of Spleen Meridian
of Foot-Taiyin,SP.)

Zuyangming Weijingxue
(points of Stomach Meridian
of Foot-Yangming,ST.)

内踝 malleolus medialis

4   **Fig. 3 The osseous and muscular landmarks on the anterior surface of the body**

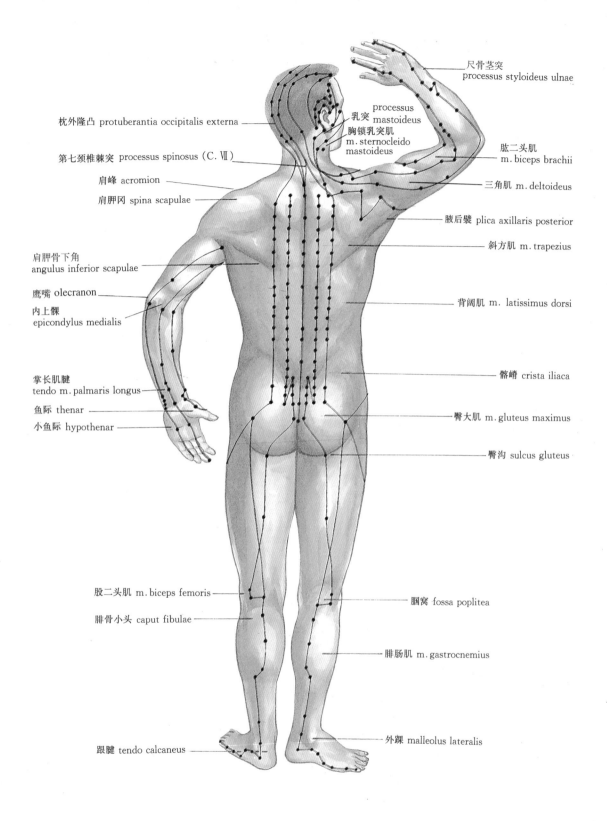

枕外隆凸 protuberantia occipitalis externa

第七颈椎棘突 processus spinosus（C.Ⅶ）

肩峰 acromion

肩胛冈 spina scapulae

肩胛骨下角
angulus inferior scapulae

鹰嘴 olecranon

内上髁
epicondylus medialis

掌长肌腱
tendo m. palmaris longus

鱼际 thenar

小鱼际 hypothenar

股二头肌 m. biceps femoris

腓骨小头 caput fibulae

跟腱 tendo calcaneus

尺骨茎突
processus styloideus ulnae

processus
乳突 mastoideus

胸锁乳突肌
m. sternocleido
mastoideus

肱二头肌
m. biceps brachii

三角肌 m. deltoideus

腋后襞 plica axillaris posterior

斜方肌 m. trapezius

背阔肌 m. latissimus dorsi

髂嵴 crista iliaca

臀大肌 m. gluteus maximus

臀沟 sulcus gluteus

腘窝 fossa poplitea

腓肠肌 m. gastrocnemius

外踝 malleolus lateralis

Fig. 4 The osseous and muscular landmarks on the posterior surface of the body　　5

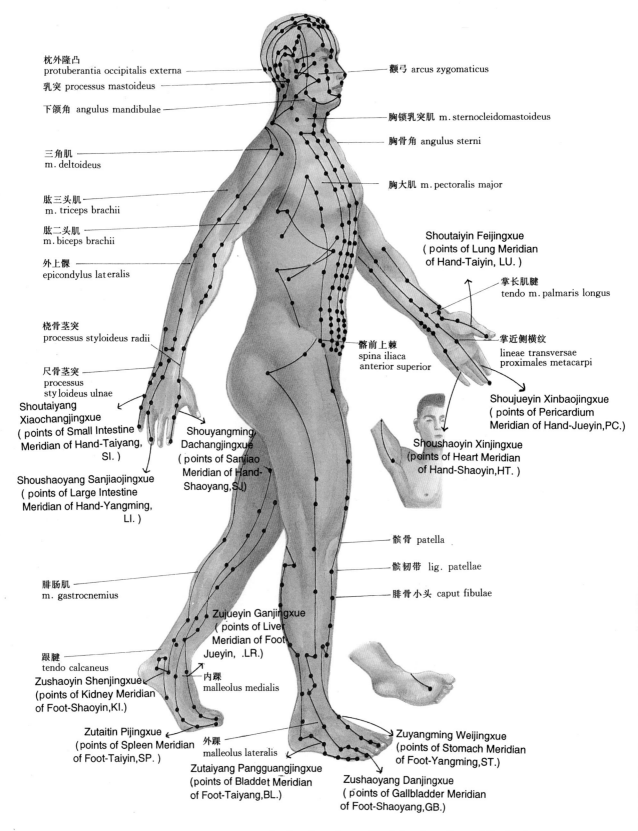

枕外隆凸 protuberantia occipitalis externa

乳突 processus mastoideus

下颌角 angulus mandibulae

三角肌 m. deltoideus

肱三头肌 m. triceps brachii

肱二头肌 m. biceps brachii

外上髁 epicondylus lateralis

桡骨茎突 processus styloideus radii

尺骨茎突 processus styloideus ulnae

Shoutaiyang Xiaochangjingxue (points of Small Intestine Meridian of Hand-Taiyang, SI.)

Shoushaoyang Sanjiaojingxue (points of Large Intestine Meridian of Hand-Yangming, LI.)

腓肠肌 m. gastrocnemius

跟腱 tendo calcaneus

Zushaoyin Shenjingxue (points of Kidney Meridian of Foot-Shaoyin,KI.)

Zutaitin Pijingxue (points of Spleen Meridian of Foot-Taiyin,SP.)

颧弓 arcus zygomaticus

胸锁乳突肌 m. sternocleidomastoideus

胸骨角 angulus sterni

胸大肌 m. pectoralis major

Shoutaiyin Feijingxue (points of Lung Meridian of Hand-Taiyin, LU.)

掌长肌腱 tendo m. palmaris longus

掌近侧横纹 lineae transversae proximales metacarpi

髂前上棘 spina iliaca anterior superior

Shoujueyin Xinbaojingxue (points of Pericardium Meridian of Hand-Jueyin,PC.)

Shoushaoyin Xinjingxue (points of Heart Meridian of Hand-Shaoyin,HT.)

髌骨 patella

髌韧带 lig. patellae

腓骨小头 caput fibulae

Zujueyin Ganjingxue (points of Liver Meridian of Foot-Jueyin, .LR.)

内踝 malleolus medialis

外踝 malleolus lateralis

Zutaiyang Pangguangjingxue (points of Bladdet Meridian of Foot-Taiyang,BL.)

Zuyangming Weijingxue (points of Stomach Meridian of Foot-Yangming,ST.)

Zushaoyang Danjingxue (points of Gallbladder Meridian of Foot-Shaoyang,GB.)

Shouyangming Dachangjingxue (points of Sanjiao Meridian of Hand-Shaoyang,SJ)

6   **Fig. 5 The osseous and muscular landmarks on the lateral surface of the body**

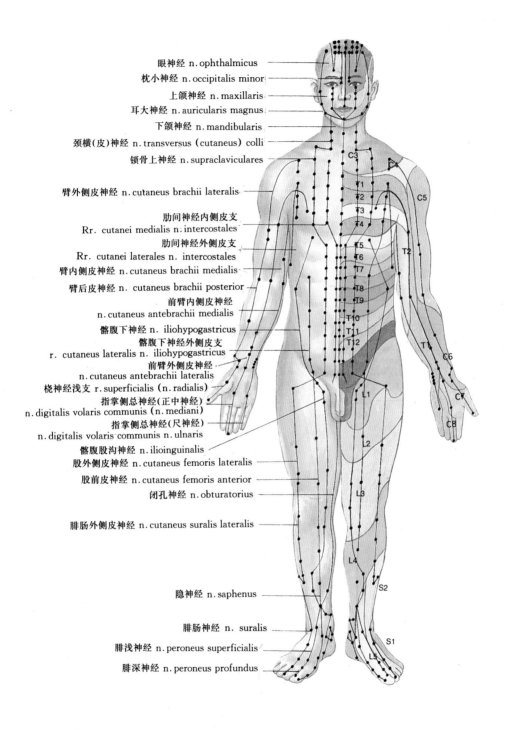

眼神经 n. ophthalmicus
枕小神经 n. occipitalis minor
上颌神经 n. maxillaris
耳大神经 n. auricularis magnus
下颌神经 n. mandibularis
颈横（皮）神经 n. transversus (cutaneus) colli
锁骨上神经 n. supraclaviculares

臂外侧皮神经 n. cutaneus brachii lateralis

肋间神经内侧皮支
Rr. cutanei medialis n. intercostales
肋间神经外侧皮支
Rr. cutanei laterales n. intercostales
臂内侧皮神经 n. cutaneus brachii medialis
臂后皮神经 n. cutaneus brachii posterior
前臂内侧皮神经
n. cutaneus antebrachii medialis
髂腹下神经 n. iliohypogastricus
髂腹下神经外侧皮支
r. cutaneus lateralis n. iliohypogastricus
前臂外侧皮神经
n. cutaneus antebrachii lateralis
桡神经浅支 r. superficialis (n. radialis)
指掌侧总神经(正中神经)
n. digitalis volaris communis (n. mediani)
指掌侧总神经(尺神经)
n. digitalis volaris communis n. ulnaris
髂腹股沟神经 n. ilioinguinalis
股外侧皮神经 n. cutaneus femoris lateralis
股前皮神经 n. cutaneus femoris anterior
闭孔神经 n. obturatorius

腓肠外侧皮神经 n. cutaneus suralis lateralis

隐神经 n. saphenus

腓肠神经 n. suralis

腓浅神经 n. peroneus superficialis
腓深神经 n. peroneus profundus

C3　C4　C5　T1　T2　T3　T4　T5　T6　T7　T8　T9　T10　T11　T12　L1　L2　L3　L4　C6　C7　C8　S2　S1　L5

Fig. 6 The segmental skin nerve distribution on the anterior aspect of the body

7

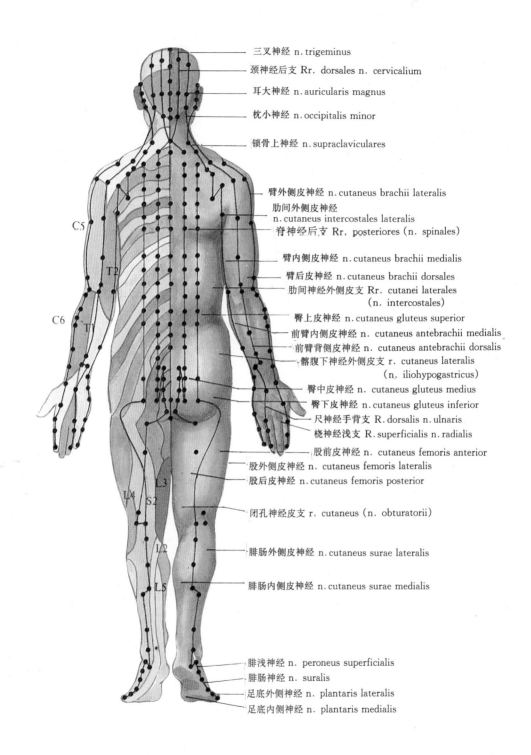

三叉神经 n. trigeminus
颈神经后支 Rr. dorsales n. cervicalium
耳大神经 n. auricularis magnus
枕小神经 n. occipitalis minor
锁骨上神经 n. supraclaviculares

臂外侧皮神经 n. cutaneus brachii lateralis
肋间外侧皮神经
n. cutaneus intercostales lateralis
脊神经后支 Rr. posteriores (n. spinales)
臂内侧皮神经 n. cutaneus brachii medialis
臂后皮神经 n. cutaneus brachii dorsales
肋间神经外侧皮支 Rr. cutanei laterales
(n. intercostales)
臀上皮神经 n. cutaneus gluteus superior
前臂内侧皮神经 n. cutaneus antebrachii medialis
前臂背侧皮神经 n. cutaneus antebrachii dorsalis
髂腹下神经外侧皮支 r. cutaneus lateralis
(n. iliohypogastricus)
臀中皮神经 n. cutaneus gluteus medius
臀下皮神经 n. cutaneus gluteus inferior
尺神经手背支 R. dorsalis n. ulnaris
桡神经浅支 R. superficialis n. radialis
股前皮神经 n. cutaneus femoris anterior
股外侧皮神经 n. cutaneus femoris lateralis
股后皮神经 n. cutaneus femoris posterior

闭孔神经皮支 r. cutaneus (n. obturatorii)

腓肠外侧皮神经 n. cutaneus surae lateralis

腓肠内侧皮神经 n. cutaneus surae medialis

腓浅神经 n. peroneus superficialis
腓肠神经 n. suralis
足底外侧神经 n. plantaris lateralis
足底内侧神经 n. plantaris medialis

C5
T2
C6
T1
L3
L4
S2
L2
L5

8   **Fig. 7 The segmental skin nerve distribution on the posterior aspect of the body**

Appendix 1
The courses, the nomenclature of the points and indications of the fourteen meridian

1. Points of Lung Meridian of Hand-Taiyin, LU

Starting from the middle *Jiao*, it runs downward to connect with the large intestine, then turns back along the cardial orifice of the stomack. It passes through the diaphragm and enters the chest to relate to the lungs, where it goes up along the trachea to the throat. It then runs toward the lateroinferior aspect to merge at Zhongfu (LU 1), which is on the latero superior aspect of the front wall of the chest. From Zhongfu, it goes along the lateral bicipital groove, passing in front of the heart meridian of Hand-Shaoyin and the pericardium meridian of Hand-Jueyin to Chize (LU 5) at the elbow. It then runs continuously down along the radial surface of the forearm and arrives at Lieque (LU 7), which lies above the styloid process of radius and between the branchioradial muscle and the long abductor muscle of the thumb. It continues along the carpalis radiale to the radial side of the palm, passing the thenar eminence to Shaoshang (LU 11), which is at the radial side of the thumb, connecting with the Large Intestine Meridian of Hand-Yangming.

This meridian has 11 points in the right and left sides from Zhongfu to Shaoshang.

Zhongfu (LU 1) Yunmen (LU 2) Tianfu (LU 3) Xiabai (LU 4) Chize (LU 5) Kongzui (LU 6) Lieque (LU 7) Jingqu (LU 8) Taiyuan (LU 9) Yuji (LU 10) Shaoshang (LU 11)

Indications of this meridian: cough, asthma, hemoptysis, sore throat and other problems relating to respiration.

2. Points of Large Intestine Meridian of Hand-Yangming, LI

Starting from the radial side of the end of the index finger, it runs upward along the radial side of the posterior of the index finger and passes through the interspace of the first and second metacarpal bones, Hegu (LI 4). Then it goes into the depression between the tendons of muscle extansor *pollicis longus and brevis* to the elbow along the lateral of the forearm. From there it ascends along the lateral of the upper arm to the Jianyu (LI 15), which is at the anterior border of *acromion*. It then turns back to travel across to the cervical vertebra where it enters into the supraclavicular fossa, descending into the chest to connect with the lung. It passes through the diaphragm to the abdomen to connect with the large intestine. A branch at the supraclavicular fossa runs upward on the lateral aspect of the neck to the face, entering into the mandible and turning around the upper labium. It crosses its paired meridian through Renzhong (DU 26) to end at Yingxiang (LI 20) in the nasolabial groove on the opposite side, where it links with the Stomach Meridian of Foot-Yangming.

This meridian has 20 points in the right and left sides from Shangyang (LI 1) to Yingxiang (LI 20)

Shangyang (LI 1) Erjian (LI 2) Sanjian (LI 3) Hegu (LI 4) Yangxi (LI 5) Pianli (LI 6) Wenliu (LI 7) Xialian (LI 8) Shanglian (LI 9) Shousanli (LI 10) Quchi (LI 11) Zhouliao (LI 12) Shouwuli (LI 13) Binao (LI 14) Jianyu (LI 15) Jugu (LI 16) Tianding (LI 17) Futu (LI 18) Kouheliao (Li 19) Yingxiang (LI 20)

Indications of this meridian: disorders of the head, face, eye, nose, mouth, teeth and throat, and bebrile diseases.

3. Points of Stomach Meridian of Foot-Yangming, ST

Starting from ala nasi, it runs upwards to the radix nasi and connects with BL. Then it goes down along the lateral side of the nose to pass through Chengqi (ST 1), entering into the upper gums. It continues to run around the lips and connects in Chengjiang (RN 24), where it turns laterally to the anterior of the mandible to pass through Daying (ST 5) and Jiache (ST 6). It passes upward to the anterior of the ear to cross Xiaguan (ST 7) to point Touwei (ST 8) within the anterior hairline at the corner of the forehead. Facial branch of the ST: from Daying (ST 5) it runs down to connect with Renying (ST 9) and passes through the lateral of the throat into the supraclavicular fossa. Then it travels down into the chest, passes through the diaphragm and connects with the stomach and the spleen. The vertical branch of ST at the supraclavicular fossa: from the supraclavicular fossa it continues down to pass through the nipple and then through the lateral of the umbilicus to meet Qichong (ST 30) in the lower abdomen. The branch of ST in the pars pylorica of the stomach: it goes down inside the abdomen to meet Qichong (ST 30). Then it runs down to Biguan (ST 31) and passes through Futu (ST 32). It continues down to the anterior of the leg to the knee. From there it goes down along the lateral to the anterior crest of the tibia and passes through the ankle joint and the dorsum pedis, ending at the lateral side of the second toe. The branch of ST in anterior tibial part: leaving Zusanli (ST 36), which is 3 *cun* below the knee, it runs down along the lateral of the anterior tibia and continues down to the lateral side of the middle toe. The branch of ST in the back of the foot: leaving Chongyang (ST 42), which is between the tendons of musculus extensor hallucis longus and musculus extensor digitorum longus at the highest part of the dorsum pedis, it enters into the extremitas medialis of the hallux and links with the Spleen Meridian of Foot-Taiyin.

This meridian has 45 points in the right and left sides from Chengqi (ST 1) to Lidui (ST 45)

Chengqi (ST 1) Sibai (ST 2) Juliao (ST 3) Dicang (ST 4) Daying (ST 5) Jiache

(ST 6) Xiaguan (ST 7) Touwei (ST 8) Renying (ST 9) Shuitu (ST 10) Qishe (ST 11) Quepen (ST 12) Qihu (ST 13) Kufang (ST 14) Wuyi (ST 15) Yingchuang (ST 16) Ruzhong (ST 17) Rugen (ST 18) Burong (ST 19) Chengman (ST 20) Liangmen (ST 21) Guanmen (ST 22) Taiyi (ST 23) Huaroumen (ST 24) Tianshu (ST 25) Wailing (ST 26) Daju (ST 27) Shuidao (ST 28) Guilai (ST 29) Qichong (ST 30) Biguan (ST 31) Futu (ST 32) Yinshi (ST 33) Liangqiu (ST 34) Dubi (ST 35) Zusanli (ST 36) Shangjuxu (ST 37) Tiaokou (ST 38) Xiajuxu (ST 39) Fenglong (ST 40) Jiexi (ST 41) Chongyang (ST 42) Xianggu (ST 43) Neiting (ST 44) Lidui (ST 45)

Indications of this meridian: disorders of the head, face, mouth, teeth, throat, stomach and intestines and blood, febrile diseases and unconsciousness.

4. Points of Spleen Meridian of Foot-Taiyin, SP

Starting from the extremitas medialis of the hallux, it runs along the medial aspect of the hallux and ascends in front of the medial malleolus up to the tibia. It follows the rear of the medial aspect of the tibia and passes through the medial aspect of the leg to Chongmen (SP 12), which is at the lateral side of the inguin. It then goes into the cavitas abdominis to pass into the spleen, connecting with the stomach. It then continues to cross the diaphragm into the chest and ascends along the esophagus and the lateral sides of the pharynx to the root of the tongue and spreads over its lower surface. The stomach branch: it traverses the diaphragm to link with the heart and connects with the Heart Meridian of Hand-Shaoyin.

This meridian has 21 points in the right and left sides from Yinbai (SP 1) to Dabao (SP 21).

Yinbai (SP 1) Dadu (SP 2) Taibai (SP 3) Gongsun (SP 4) Shangqiu (SP 5) Sanyinjiao (SP 6) Lougu (SP 7) Diji (SP 8) Yinlingquan (SP 9) Xuehai (SP 10) Jimen (SP 11) Chongmen (SP 12) Fushe (SP 13) Fujie (SP 14) Daheng (SP 15) Fu'ai (SP 16) Shidou (SP 17) Tianxi (SP 18) Xiongxiang (SP 19) Zhourong (SP 20) Dabao (SP 21)

Indications of this meridian: disorders of the spleen, stomach, heart, lung, reproductive and urinary organs.

5. Points of Heart Meridian of Hand-Shaoyin, HT

Starting from the heart, the descending branch runs down to pass through the diaphragm into the cavitas abdominis to spread over the small intestine. The ascending branch: it runs alongside the esophagus from the heart to pass through the collum into the brain to link with the ocular connectors. The rectilinear branch of the HT: from the heart to the lung it traverses laterally to Jiquan (HT 1), which is at the top point of the axilla. From there it goes along the postero-medial aspect of the upper arm and passes alongside the posterior of the Lung Meridian of Hand-Taiyin and the Pericardium Meridian of Hand-Jueyin to point Shaohai (ST 3). This is at the center of the connecting line between the extremitas medialis of the cubital fossa and the medial epicondyle of humerus. From there it continues along the postero-medial aspect of the forearm to the pisiform region proximal to the palm and enters the palm. Then it runs along the radial border of the little finger and connects with the Small Intestine Meridian of Hand-Taiyang.

This meridian has 9 points in the right and left sides from Jiquan (HT 1) to Shaochong (HT 9).

Jiquan (HT 1) Qingling (HT 2) Shaohai (HT 3) Lingdao (HT 4) Tongli (HT 5) Yinxi (HT 6) Shenmen (HT 7) Shaofu (HT 8) Shaochong (HT 9)

Indications of this meridian: unconsciousness, blood disorders, dry throat, thirst, jaudice, hypochondriac pain, precordial pain and pain along the medial aspect of the upper arm.

6. Points of Small Intestine Meridian of Hand-Taiyang, SI

Starting from the ulnar side of the little finger, it runs up along the lateral side of the dorsum of the hand to the wrist and passes through the styloid process of the ulnar. From there it goes up along the posterior border of the lateral aspect of the forearm and passes between the olecranon and medial epicondyle of the humerus. Then it passes along the posterior border of the lateral aspect of the upper arm to the shoulder joint and continues to go around the scapular region to meet with point Dazhui (DU 14) of the Du Meridian in the upper back. From there it runs anteroinferiorly into the supraclavicular fossa and continues to enter into the heart. It runs down alongside the esophagus to cross the diaphragm and enters the cavitas abdominis to spread over the stomach and the small intestine. The branch in the supraclavicular fossa: it passes vertically up along the pars cervicalis to the facio-bucca and then through the paropia into the ear. The branch in the bucca: it runs up along the infraorbital region to pass the nasal margin to the inner canthus and connects with the Bladder Meridian of Foot-Taiyang.

This meridian has 19 points in the right and left sides from Shaoze (SI 1) to Tinggong (ST 19).

Shaoze (SI 1) Qiangu (SI 2) Houxi (SI 3) Wangu (SI 4) Yanggu (SI 5) Yanglao (SI 6) Zhizheng (SI 7) Xiaohai (SI 8) Jianzhen (SI 9) Naoshu (SI 10) Tianzong (SI 11) Bingfeng (SI 12) Quyan (SI 13) Jianwaishu (SI 14) Jianzhongshu (SI 15) Tianchuang (SI 16) Tianrong (SI 17) Quanliao (SI 18) Tinggong (SI 19)

Indications of this meridian: lower abdominial pain, lumbago, deafness, jaundice, swelling of the bucca, sore throat, and pain along the posterior of the shoulder and arm.

7. Points of Bladder Meridian of Foot-Taiyang, BL

Starting from the inner canthus, it ascends to the forehead and vertex to connect with the point Baihui (DU 20). The vertex branch: from the vertex into the pars intracranialis to communicate with the brain, it emerges from the brain to travel down along the nape. It then passes through the medial border of the scapula, which is 1.5 *cun* from the midline, and continues along the lateral side of the spine to the lumbus. From Shenshu (BL 23) it passes through the musculi dorsi to enter the cavitas abdominis and spreads over the kidney and the bladder. The branch in the lumbus: it runs down into the popliteal fossa from the buttocks. The branch in the nape runs vertically down along the lateral side of the spine, which is 3 *cun* from the midline, and passes along the medial border of the scapula. It continues vertically downward to the lumbus and the buttocks. From there it passes along the lateral side of the posterior of the leg to meet with the branch in the lumbus in the popiteal fossa. It continues down along the superficial surface of the triceps muscle of the calf and passes along the posterior of the lateral malleolous. Finally it continues along the lateral margin of the foot to the lateral side of the little toe, where it connects with the Kidney Meridian of Foot-Shaoyin.

This meridian has 67 points in the right and left sides from Jingming (BL 1) to Zhiyin (BL 67).

Jingming (BL 1) Cuanzhu (BL 2) Meichong (BL 3) Qucha (BL 4) Wuchu (BL 5) Chengguang (BL 6) Tongtian (BL 7) Luoque (BL 8) Yuzhen (BL 9) Tianzhu (BL 10) Dazhu (BL 11) Fengmen (BL 12) Feishu (BL 13) Jueyinshu (BL 14) Xinshu (BL 15) Dushu (BL 16) Geshu (BL 17) Ganshu (BL 18) Danshu (BL 19) Pishu (Bl 20) Weishu (BL 21) Sanjiaoshu (BL 22) Shenshu (23) Qihaishu (BL 24) Dachangshu (BL 25) Guanyuanshu (BL 26) Xiaochangshu (BL 27) Pangguangshu (BL 28) Zhonglushu (BL 29) Baihuanshu (BL 30) Shangliao (BL 31) Ciliao (BL 32) Zhongliao (BL 33) Xialiao (Bl 34) Huiyang (BL 35) Chengfu (BL 36) Yinmen (BL 37) Fuxi (BL 38) Weiyang (BL 39) Weizhong (BL 40) Fufen (BL 41) Pohu (BL 42) Gaohuang (BL 43) Shentang (BL 44) Yixi (BL 45) Geguan (BL 46) Hunmen (BL 47) Yanggang (BL 48) Yishe (BL 49) Weicang (BL 50) Huangmen (BL 51) Zhishi (BL 52) Baohuang (BL 53) Zhibian (BL 54) Heyang (BL 55) Chengjin (BL 56) Chengshan (BL 57) Feiyang (BL 58) Fuyang (BL 59) Kunlun (BL 60) Pucan (BL 61) Shenmai (BL 62) Jinmen (BL 63) Jinggu (BL 64) Shugu (BL 65) Zutonggu (BL 66) Zhiyin (BL 67)

Indications of this meridian: disorders of the head, nape, eye, dorso-lumbar region and leg, and uncounsciousness. The points in the first and second adjacent lines parallel to the spine can treat the diseases related to the Zang-Fu.

8. Points of Kidney Meridian of Foot-Shaoyin, KI

Starting from the inferior aspect of the fifth toe, it runs obliquely to the sole and then passes the posterior of the medial malleolus to the heel. It continues upward along the posterior border of the medial side of the tibia, passing the medial side of the popliteal fossa to the posterior-medial aspect of the thigh. It then passes the spine and enters the cavitas abdominis, where it connects with the kidney and bladder. The straight branch in the kidney: it runs upward from the kidney to pass through the liver and diaphragm and then enters the chest to link with the lung. It continues alongside the trachea and the throat and terminates at the root of the tongue. The branch in the lung: it goes to the heart from the lung and spreads over the chest to connect with the Pericardium Meridian of Hand-Jueyin.

This meridian has 27 points in the right and left sides from Yongquan (KI 1) to Shufu (KI 27).

Yongquan (KI 1) Rangu (KI 2) Taixi (KI 3) Dazhong (KI 4) Shuiquan (KI 5) Zhaohai (KI 6) Fuliu (KI 7) Jiaoxin (KI 8) Zhubin (KI 9) Yingu (KI 10) Henggu (KI 11) Dahe (KI 12) Qixue (KI 13) Siman (KI 14) Zhongzhu (KI 15) Huangshu (KI 16) Shangqu (KI 17) Shiguan (KI 18) Yindu (KI 19) Futonggu (KI 20) Youmen (KI 21) Bulang (KI 22) Shenfeng (KI 23) Lingxu (KI 24) Shencang (KI 25) Yuzhong (KI 26) Shufu (KI 27)

Indications of this meridian: gynecopathy, disorders of kidney, bladder, lung, spleen and liver.

9. Points of Pericardium Meridian of Hand-Jueyin, PC

Starting from the chest, it enters the pericardium and descends through the diaphragm to the cavitas abdominis. It connects, successively, with the upper, middle and lower Jiao from the chest to the abdomen. The chest branch: it emerges from the chest at a point 5 *cun* lateral to the midline in the fourth intercostal space, Tianchi (PC 1). Then it runs along the midline of the medial aspect of the upper arm, passing down between the Lung Meridian of Hand-Taiyin and the Heart Meridian of Hand-Shaoyin to the cubital fossa. It continues along the palmar aspect of the forearm and passes the middle of the wrist to enter the palm, ending in the tip of middle finger. The branch in the palm: it sets apart from the Laogong (PC 8) and runs along the ring finger to the tip of the forth finger, where it links with the Sanjiao Meridian of Hand-Shaoyang.

This meridian has 9 points in the right and left sides from Tianchi (PC 1) to Zhongchong (PC 9).

Tianchi (PC 1) Tianquan (PC 2) Quze (PC 3) Ximen (PC 4) Jianshi (PC 5) Neiguan (PC 6) Daling (PC 7) Laogong (PC 8) Zhongchong (PC 9)

Indications of this meridian: disorders of heart, chest, stomach, skin, mouth, including angina pectoris (pain in chest), and hypochondric region and unconsciousness.

10. Points of Sanjiao Meridian of Hand-Shaoyang, SJ

Starting from the tip of the dorsal aspect of the ring finger, it runs up between the fourth and fifth metacarpal bones along the dorsum of the hand and passes along the dorsum of the forearm between the radius and the ulna to the elbow. From there it runs along the lateral aspect of the upper arm to the shoulder joint and passes anteriorly into the supraclavicular fossa. It then descends to pass the Danzhong (RN 17) point and connects with the pericardium. It continues down through the diaphragm to enter the cavitas abdominis, where it joints its pertaining organ, the upper, middle and lower Jiao, from the chest to the abdomen. The branch in the chest: it runs up from Danzhong (RN 17) into the supraclavicular fossa and goes to the neck. It passes through the nape and then behind the ear to the region directly above the ear apex. From there it curves into the infraorbital region in the faciobucca. The branch in the ear: it runs into the intra-auris from the retro-auricular region and emerges at the preauricular region to the outer canthus, where it connects with the Gallbladder Meridian of Foot-Shaoyang.

This meridian has 23 points in the right and left sides from Guanchong (SJ 1) to Sizhukong (SJ 23).

Guanchong (SJ 1) Yemen (SJ 2) Zhongzhu (SJ 3) Yangchi (SJ 4) Waiguan (SJ 5) Zhigou (SJ 6) Huizong (SJ 7) Sanyanglou (SJ 8) Sidu (SJ 9) Tianjing (SJ 10) Qinglengyuan (SJ 11) Xiaolou (SJ 12) Naohui (SJ 13) Jianliao (SJ 14) Tianliao (SJ 15) Tianyou (SJ 16) Yifeng (SJ 17) Chimai (SJ 18) Luxi (SJ 19) Jiaosun (SJ 20) Ermen (SJ 21) Erheliao (SJ 22) Sizhukong (SJ 23)

Indications of this meridian: headache, dizziness, deafness, sore throat, febrile diseases and unconsciousness.

11. Points of Gallbladder Meridian of Foot-Shaoyang, GB

Starting from the outer canthus, it runs laterally to the preauricular region and goes up to the frontal angle. From there it continues inferiorly and poteriorly behind the ear to reach the Wangu (GB 12) point, where it reverses its direction passing anteriorly to Yangbai (GB 14) at the forehead. It then reverses its direction once more posteriorly and inferiorly to Jianjing (GB 21), passing through the neck into the supraclavicular fossa. The branch in the ear: it runs into the intro-auris from the retro-auricular region and emerges from the preauricular region to the posterior aspect of the outer canthus. The branch in outer canthus: it runs to the infraorbital region from the outer canthus and passes through the Jiache (ST 6) and neck into the supraclavicular fossa to meet the former branch. It then descends into the chest and passes through the diaphragm into the cavitas abdominis to connect with the liver and gallbladder. It runs down along the interior of the abdominal wall to the vulva region where it emerges from the abdominal wall. It passes through the inguinal region to the Huantiao (GB 30). The straight branch in the supraclavicular fossa: from the anterior of the axillary fossa it runs down along the lateral aspect of the chest to meet the branch which enters into Huantiao (GB 30). It then continues down along the lateral aspect of the leg to the knee and down along the lateral aspect of the fibula to the anterior region of the lateral malleolus. It passes through the dorsum of the foot to the lateral side of the fourth toe. The branch in the dorsum of the foot: it springs from Zulinqi (GB 41) and runs medially to the distal portion of the great toe where it connects with the Liver Meridian of Foot-Jueyin.

This meridian has 44 points in the right and left sides from Tongziliao (GB 1) to Zuqiaoyin (GB 44).

Tongziliao (GB 1) Tinghui (GB 2) Shangguan (GB 3) Hanyan (GB 4) Xuanlu (GB 5) Xuanli (GB 6) Qubin (GB 7) Shuaigu (GB 8) Tianchong (GB 9) Fubai (GB 10) Touqiaoyin (GB 11) Wangu (GB 12) Benshen (GB 13) Yangbai (Gb 14) Toulinqi (GB 15) Muchuang (GB 16) Zhengying (Gb 17) Chengling (Gb 18) Naokong (GB 19) Fenchi (GB 20) Jianjing (GB 21) Yuanye (GB 22) Zhejin (GB

23) Riyue (GB 24) Jingmen (GB 25) Daimai (GB 26) Wushu (GB 27) Weidao (GB 28) Juliao (GB 29) Huantiao (GB 30) Fengshi (GB 31) Zhongdu (GB 32) Xiyangguan (GB 33) Yanglingquan (GB 34) Yangjiao (GB 35) Waiqiu (GB 36) Guangming (GB 37) Yangfu (GB 38) Xuanzhong (GB 39) Qiuxu (GB 40) Zulinqi (GB 41) Diwuhui (GB 42) Xiaxi (GB 43) Zuqiaoyin (GB 44)

The indications of this meridian: disorders of lateral aspect of head, eye, ear, chest and hypochondrium, febrile diseases and gynecopathy.

12. Points of Liver Meridian of Foot-Jueyin, LR

Originating from the great toe, it runs upwards along the dorsum of the foot and passes in front of the medial malleolus to Zhongfeng (LR 4). From there it ascends along the medial aspect of the tibia to the medial region of the knee and passes through the medial aspect of the thigh. It travels around the vulva to enter the cavitas abdominis where it spreads over the liver and the gallbladder. It then passes through the diaphragm and ascends along the chest wall. It continues to pass through the posterior of the throat into the nasal cavity where it connects with the visual organ and meets the Du Meridian at the vertex. The branch from the visual organ: it runs downward from the visual organ into the facio-bucca and around the lip. The branch from the liver: it sets out from the liver and passes through the diaphragm into the chest. It connects with the lung, linking with the Lung Meridian of Hand-Taiyin.

This meridian has 14 points in the right and left sides from Dadun (LR 1) to Qimen (LR 14).

Dadun (LR 1) Xingjian (LR 2) Taichong (LR 3) Zhongfeng (LR 4) Ligou (LR 5) Zhongdu (LR 6) Xiguan (LR 7) Ququan (LR 8) Yinbao (LR 9) Zuwuli (LR 10) Yinlian (LR 11) Jimai (LR 12) Zhangmen (LR 13) Qimen (LR 14)

The indications of this meridian: hepatopathy, gynecopathy, diseases of external genitalia, and disorders of gallbladder, kidney, heart, spleen and lung.

13. Points of Du Meridian, DU

It starts from inside the pelvis and descends to emerge from the perineum. Then it runs upward along the interior of the spinal column and passes through the dorsum of the neck where it enters the brain. It continues sagittally over the vertex and forehead and passes through the columella of the nose and Shuigou (DU 26), which is in the upper lip. It ends at the frenulum of the upper lip.

This meridian has 28 points from Changqiang (DU 1) to Yinjiao (DU 28).

Changqiang (DU 1) Yaoshu (DU 2) Yaoyangguan (DU 3) Mingmen (DU 4) Xuanshu (DU 5) Jizhong (DU 6) Zhongshu (DU 7) Jinsuo (DU 8) Zhiyang (DU 9) Lingtai (DU 10) Shendao (DU 11) Shenzhu (DU 12) Taodao (DU 13) Dazhui (DU 14) Yamen (DU 15) Fengfu (DU 16) Naohu (DU 17) Qiangjian (DU 18) Houding (DU 19) Baihui (DU 20) Qianding (DU 21) Xinhui (DU 22) Shangxing (DU 23) Shenting (DU 24) Suliao (DU 25) Shuigou (DU 26) Duiduan (DU 27) Yinjiao (DU 28)

The indications of this meridian: dizziness, manicdepressive psychosis, stroke, febrile diseases and the need for emergency treatment.

14. Points of Ren Meridian, RN

It arises from the pelvis and emerges from the perineum. It ascends along the mons pubis and the midline of the abdomen and passes through the chest to the laryngeal protuberance. From there it arrives at the lower lip and curves around the lips where it continues upwards into the infraorbital region.

This meridian has 24 points from Huiyin (RN 1) to Chengjiang (RN 24)

Huiyin (RN 1) Qugu (RN 2) Zhongji (RN 3) Guanyuan (RN 4) Shimen (RN 5) Qihai (RN 6) Yinjiao (RN 7) Shenque (RN 8) Shuifen (RN 9) Xiawan (RN 10) Jianli (RN 11) Zhongwan (RN 12) Shangwan (RN 13) Juque (RN 14) Jiuwei (RN 15) Zhongting (RN 16) Danzhong (RN 17) Yutang (RN 18) Zigong (RN 19) Huagai (RN 20) Xuanji (RN 21) Tiantu (RN 22) Lianquan (RN 23) Chengjiang (RN 24)

The indications of this meridian: disorders of liver, kidney, spleen, stomach, heart, lung and throat.

Part 2

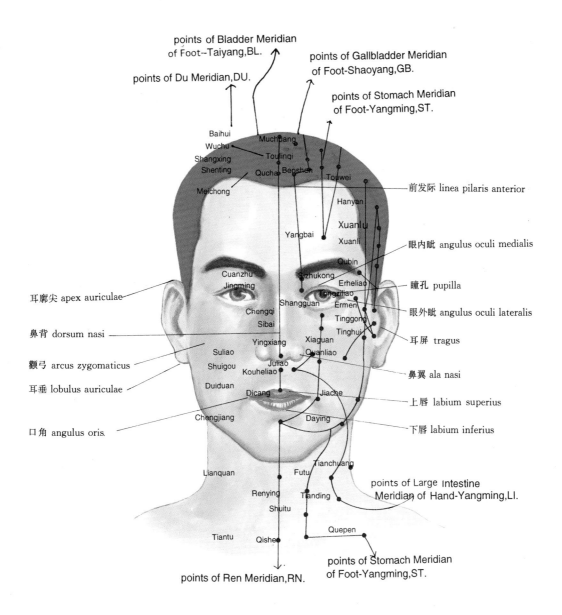

points of Bladder Meridian of Foot--Taiyang,BL.

points of Gallbladder Meridian of Foot-Shaoyang,GB.

points of Du Meridian,DU.

points of Stomach Meridian of Foot-Yangming,ST.

Baihui
Wuchu
Muchuang
Shangxing
Toulinqi
Shenting
Qucha
Benshen
Meichong
Touwei

前发际 linea pilaris anterior

Hanyan

Xuanlu

Yangbai
Xuanli

眼内眦 angulus oculi medialis

Qubin

Cuanzhu
Sizhukong
Erheliao

瞳孔 pupilla

Jingming
Tongziliao

耳廓尖 apex auriculae
Shangguan
Ermen

眼外眦 angulus oculi lateralis

Chengqi
Tinggong
Sibai
Tinghui

耳屏 tragus

鼻背 dorsum nasi
Yingxiang
Xiaguan

颧弓 arcus zygomaticus
Suliao
Quanliao

鼻翼 ala nasi

Shuigou
Juliao

耳垂 lobulus auriculae
Kouheliao

上唇 labium superius

Duiduan
Dicang
Jiache

下唇 labium inferius

Chengjiang
Daying

口角 angulus oris

Tianchuang

Lianquan
Futu
points of Large Intestine Meridian of Hand-Yangming,LI.

Renying
Tianding

Shuitu

Quepen

Tiantu
Qishe

points of Stomach Meridian of Foot-Yangming,ST.

points of Ren Meridian,RN.

Fig. 8 The skin and points on the craniofacial region

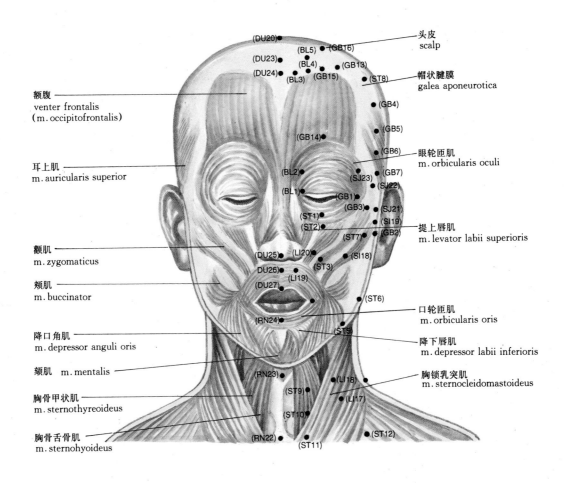

Fig. 9 The muscles and points on the craniofacial region

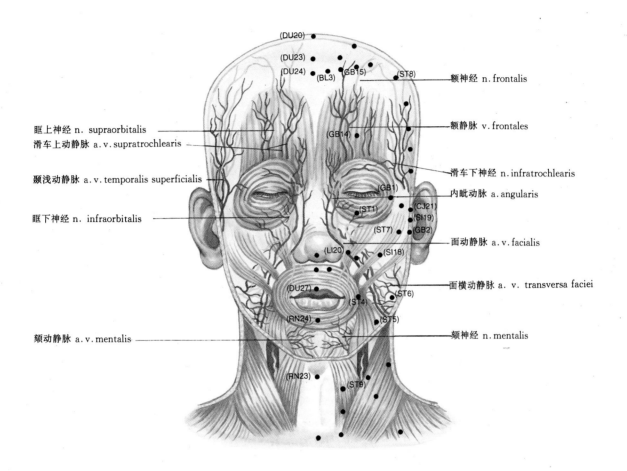

Fig. 10 The blood vessels, nerves and points on the craniofacial region 23

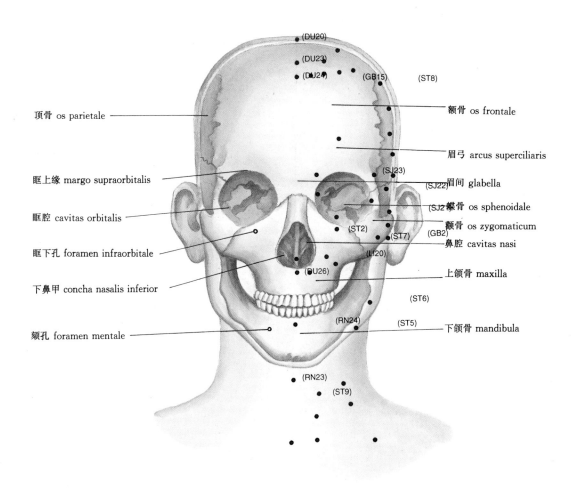

顶骨 os parietale

眶上缘 margo supraorbitalis

眶腔 cavitas orbitalis

眶下孔 foramen infraorbitale

下鼻甲 concha nasalis inferior

颏孔 foramen mentale

(DU20)
(DU23)
(DU24)
(GB15)
(ST8)
额骨 os frontale

眉弓 arcus superciliaris

(SJ23)
眉间 glabella (SJ22)

蝶骨 os sphenoidale (SJ2)

颧骨 os zygomaticum

(ST2)
(ST7) (GB2)

鼻腔 cavitas nasi

(LI20)

上颌骨 maxilla

(DU26)

(ST6)

(RN24)
(ST5)
下颌骨 mandibula

(RN23)
(ST9)

Fig. 11 The skeleton and points on the craniofacial region

24

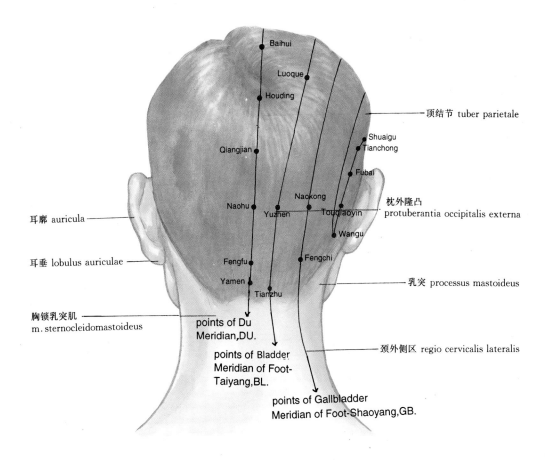

Baihui

Luoque

Houding

顶结节 tuber parietale

Shuaigu
Tianchong

Qiangjian

Fubai

Naokong

耳廓 auricula

Naohu

Yuzhen

Touqiaoyin

枕外隆凸
protuberantia occipitalis externa

Wangu

耳垂 lobulus auriculae

Fengfu

Fengchi

Yamen

乳突 processus mastoideus

Tianzhu

胸锁乳突肌
m. sternocleidomastoideus

points of Du
Meridian,DU.

颈外侧区 regio cervicalis lateralis

points of Bladder
Meridian of Foot-
Taiyang,BL.

points of Gallbladder
Meridian of Foot-Shaoyang,GB.

Fig. 12 The skin and points on the posterior of head

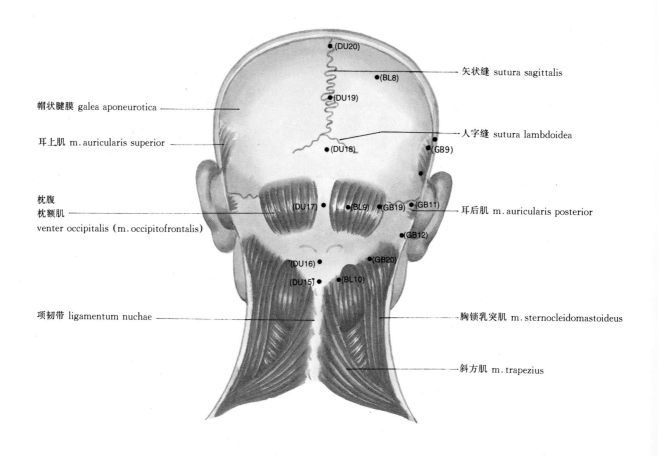

帽状腱膜 galea aponeurotica

耳上肌 m.auricularis superior

枕腹
枕额肌
venter occipitalis（m.occipitofrontalis）

项韧带 ligamentum nuchae

(DU20)
(BL8)
(DU19)
(DU18)
(GB9)
矢状缝 sutura sagittalis
人字缝 sutura lambdoidea
(DU17) (BL9) (GB19) (GB11)
(GB12)
耳后肌 m.auricularis posterior
(DU16) (GB20)
(DU15) (BL10)
胸锁乳突肌 m.sternocleidomastoideus
斜方肌 m.trapezius

26 **Fig. 13 The muscles and points on the posterior of head**

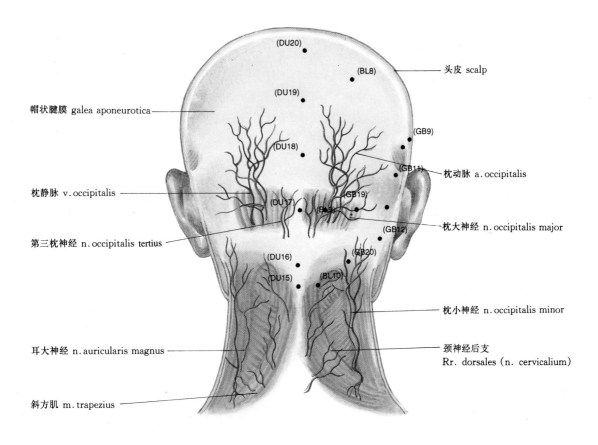

(DU20)

(BL8)

头皮 scalp

(DU19)

帽状腱膜 galea aponeurotica

(DU18)

(GB9)

(GB11)

枕动脉 a.occipitalis

枕静脉 v.occipitalis

(GB19)

(DU17)

(GB12)

枕大神经 n.occipitalis major

第三枕神经 n.occipitalis tertius

(GB20)

(DU16)

(DU15)

(BL10)

枕小神经 n.occipitalis minor

耳大神经 n.auricularis magnus

颈神经后支
Rr. dorsales（n. cervicalium）

斜方肌 m.trapezius

Fig. 14 The blood vessels, nerves and points on the posterior of head

27

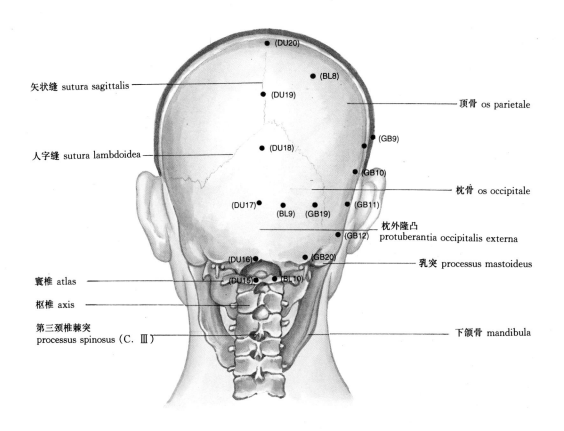

矢状缝 sutura sagittalis

人字缝 sutura lambdoidea

顶骨 os parietale

枕骨 os occipitale

枕外隆凸
protuberantia occipitalis externa

乳突 processus mastoideus

寰椎 atlas

枢椎 axis

第三颈椎棘突
processus spinosus（C. Ⅲ）

下颌骨 mandibula

(DU20)
(BL8)
(DU19)
(GB9)
(DU18)
(GB10)
(DU17)
(GB11)
(BL9) (GB19)
(GB12)
(DU16)
(GB20)
(DU15) (BL10)

28

Fig. 15 The skeleton and points on the posterior of head

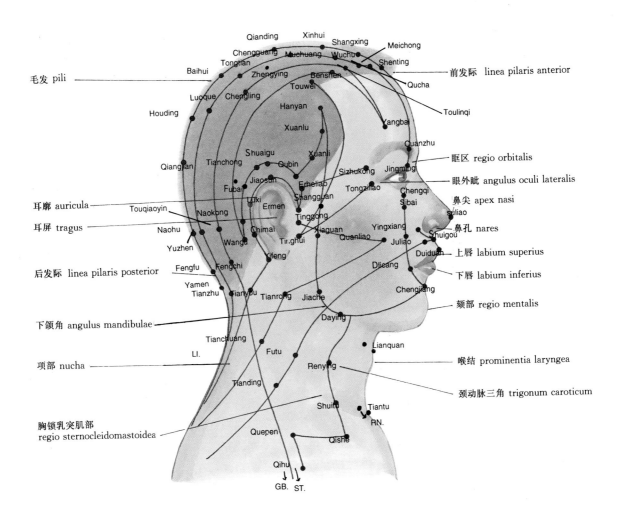

Fig. 16 The skin and points on the right aspect of the cephalocervix

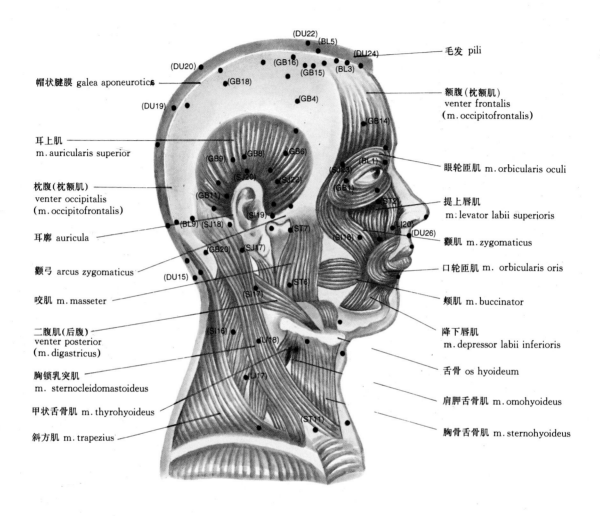

帽状腱膜 galea aponeurotica

耳上肌 m. auricularis superior

枕腹(枕额肌)
venter occipitalis
(m. occipitofrontalis)

耳廓 auricula

颧弓 arcus zygomaticus

咬肌 m. masseter

二腹肌(后腹)
venter posterior
(m. digastricus)

胸锁乳突肌
m. sternocleidomastoideus

甲状舌骨肌 m. thyrohyoideus

斜方肌 m. trapezius

毛发 pili

额腹(枕额肌)
venter frontalis
(m. occipitofrontalis)

眼轮匝肌 m. orbicularis oculi

提上唇肌
m. levator labii superioris

颧肌 m. zygomaticus

口轮匝肌 m. orbicularis oris

颊肌 m. buccinator

降下唇肌
m. depressor labii inferioris

舌骨 os hyoideum

肩胛舌骨肌 m. omohyoideus

胸骨舌骨肌 m. sternohyoideus

(DU22) (BL5) (DU24)
(GB16) (GB15) (BL3)
(GB18) (DU20)
(GB4)
(DU19)
(GB14)
(GB9) (GB8) (GB6) (BL1)
(SJ20) (SJ23)
(GB11) (SJ22) (GB1)
(SI19) (ST2)
(BL9) (SJ18) (ST7) (LI20) (DU26)
(GB20) (SJ17) (SI18)
(DU15)
(ST6)
(SI17)
(SI16)
(LI18)
(LI17)
(ST11)

30　　　**Fig. 17 The muscles and points on the right aspect of the cephalocervix**

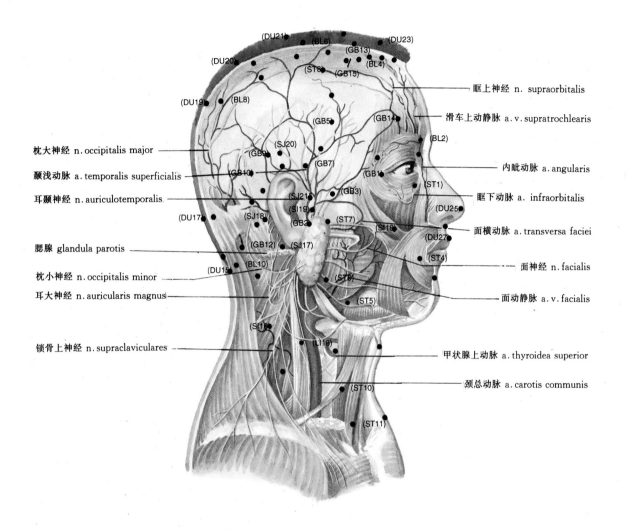

枕大神经 n. occipitalis major
颞浅动脉 a. temporalis superficialis
耳颞神经 n. auriculotemporalis

腮腺 glandula parotis

枕小神经 n. occipitalis minor
耳大神经 n. auricularis magnus

锁骨上神经 n. supraclaviculares

眶上神经 n. supraorbitalis
滑车上动静脉 a. v. supratrochlearis

内眦动脉 a. angularis
眶下动脉 a. infraorbitalis

面横动脉 a. transversa faciei

面神经 n. facialis
面动静脉 a. v. facialis

甲状腺上动脉 a. thyroidea superior
颈总动脉 a. carotis communis

(DU21) (BL6) (DU23)
(GB13)
(DU20) (ST8) (BL4)
(GB15)
(DU19) (BL8)
(GB5) (GB14)
(BL2)
(SJ20)
(GB9) (GB7)
(GB10) (GB1) (ST1)
(GB3) (DU25)
(SJ21)
(DU17) (SJ19) (ST7) (SI18)
(GB2) (DU27)
(GB12) (SJ17) (ST4)
(DU15) (BL10)
(ST6)
(ST5)
(SI16)
(LI18)
(ST10)
(ST11)

Fig. 18 The blood vessels, nerves and points on the right aspect of the cephalocervix   31

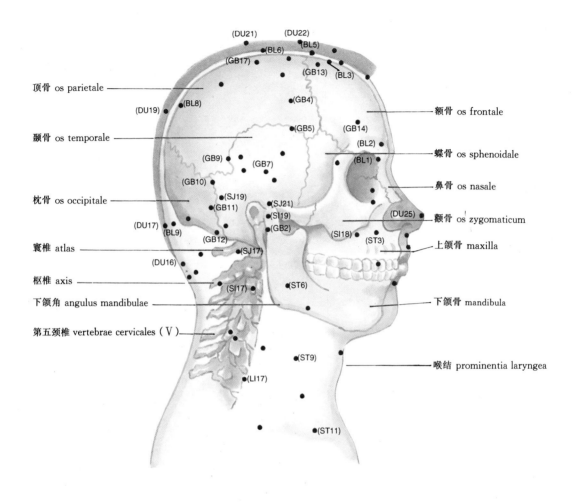

顶骨 os parietale

(DU21) (DU22)
(BL5)
(BL6)
(GB17) (GB13) (BL3)

(GB4)

(DU19) (BL8)
(GB5) (GB14)

额骨 os frontale

颞骨 os temporale

(BL2)
(BL1)

蝶骨 os sphenoidale

鼻骨 os nasale

(GB9) (GB7)

(GB10)

枕骨 os occipitale

(SJ19) (SJ21)
(GB11) (SI19)
(DU17) (GB2)
(BL9) (SI18) (ST3)
(GB12)

(DU25) 颧骨 os zygomaticum

上颌骨 maxilla

寰椎 atlas

(SJ17)
(DU16)

枢椎 axis

(SI17) (ST6)

下颌角 angulus mandibulae

下颌骨 mandibula

第五颈椎 vertebrae cervicales（Ⅴ）

(ST9)

喉结 prominentia laryngea

(LI17)

(ST11)

Fig. 19 The skeleton and points on the right aspect of the cephalocervix

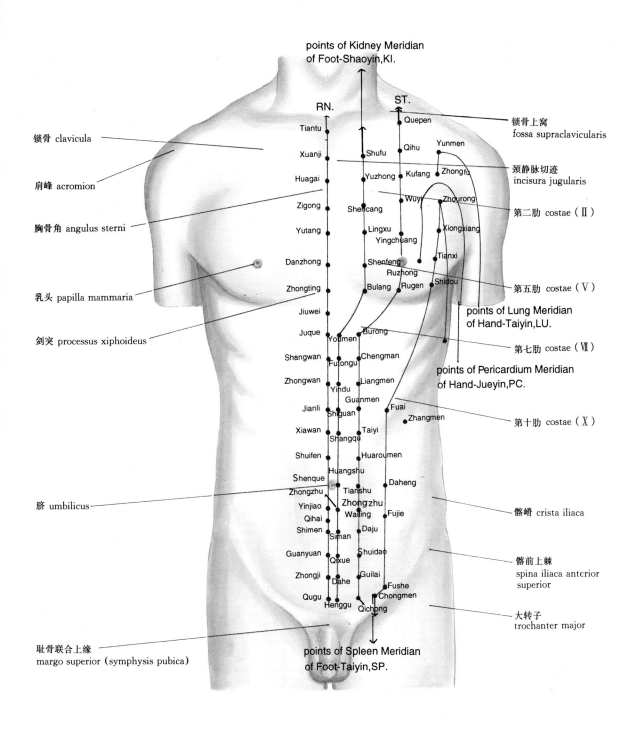

points of Kidney Meridian of Foot-Shaoyin,KI.

RN.

ST.

锁骨 clavicula

肩峰 acromion

胸骨角 angulus sterni

乳头 papilla mammaria

剑突 processus xiphoideus

脐 umbilicus

耻骨联合上缘 margo superior (symphysis pubica)

Tiantu
Xuanji
Huagai
Zigong
Yutang
Danzhong
Zhongting
Jiuwei
Juque
Shangwan
Zhongwan
Jianli
Xiawan
Shuifen
Shenque
Zhongzhu
Yinjiao
Qihai
Shimen
Guanyuan
Zhongji
Qugu
Henggu

Quepen
Qihu
Yunmen
Shufu
Yuzhong
Kufang
Zhongfu
Shencang
Wuyi
Zhourong
Lingxu
Yingchuang
Xiongxiang
Shenfeng
Tianxi
Ruzhong
Bulang
Rugen
Shidou
Burong
Youmen
Chengman
Fulongu
Liangmen
Yindu
Guanmen
Shiguan
Fuai
Taiyi
Zhangmen
Shangqu
Huaroumen
Huangshu
Daheng
Tianshu
Zhongzhu
Wailing
Fujie
Daju
Siman
Shuidao
Qixue
Guilai
Dahe
Fushe
Chongmen
Qichong

锁骨上窝 fossa supraclavicularis

颈静脉切迹 incisura jugularis

第二肋 costae（Ⅱ）

第五肋 costae（Ⅴ）

points of Lung Meridian of Hand-Taiyin,LU.

第七肋 costae（Ⅶ）

points of Pericardium Meridian of Hand-Jueyin,PC.

第十肋 costae（Ⅹ）

髂嵴 crista iliaca

髂前上棘 spina iliaca anterior superior

大转子 trochanter major

points of Spleen Meridian of Foot-Taiyin,SP.

Fig. 20 The skin and points on the anterior aspect of the trunk

33

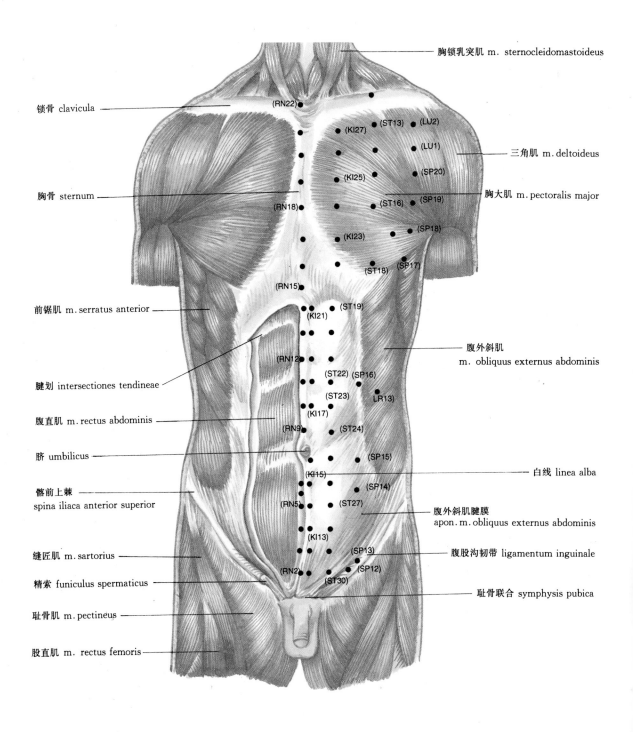

胸锁乳突肌 m. sternocleidomastoideus

锁骨 clavicula

(RN22)

(KI27) (ST13) (LU2)

(LU1)

三角肌 m. deltoideus

(KI25) (SP20)

胸骨 sternum

(RN18) (ST16) (SP19)

胸大肌 m. pectoralis major

(KI23) (SP18)

(ST18) (SP17)

(RN15)

前锯肌 m. serratus anterior

(ST19)

(KI21)

(RN12)

腹外斜肌
m. obliquus externus abdominis

(ST22) (SP16)

腱划 intersectiones tendineae

(ST23)

(LR13)

(KI17)

腹直肌 m. rectus abdominis

(RN9) (ST24)

脐 umbilicus

(SP15)

(KI15)

白线 linea alba

髂前上棘
spina iliaca anterior superior

(SP14)

(RN5) (ST27)

腹外斜肌腱膜
apon. m. obliquus externus abdominis

(KI13)

缝匠肌 m. sartorius

(SP13)

腹股沟韧带 ligamentum inguinale

精索 funiculus spermaticus

(RN2) (SP12)

(ST30)

耻骨肌 m. pectineus

耻骨联合 symphysis pubica

股直肌 m. rectus femoris

Fig. 21 The muscles and points on the anterior aspect of the trunk

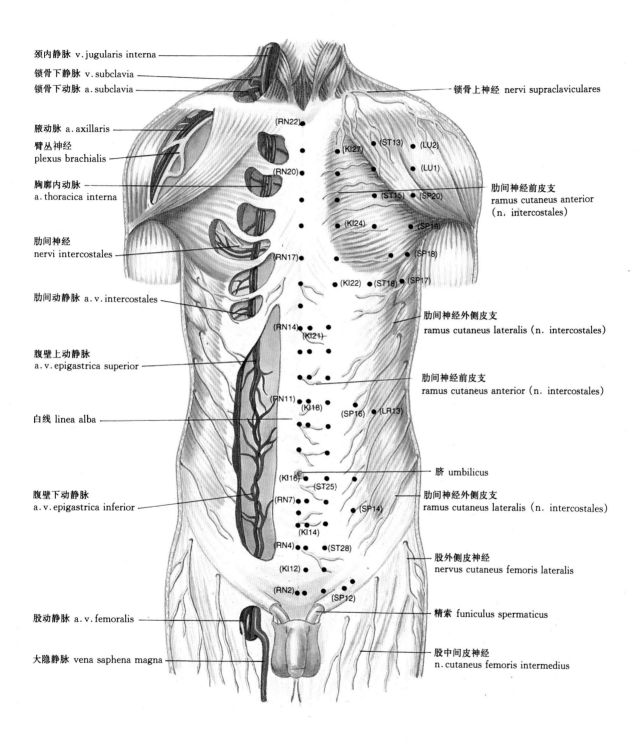

颈内静脉 v.jugularis interna

锁骨下静脉 v.subclavia

锁骨下动脉 a.subclavia

锁骨上神经 nervi supraclaviculares

腋动脉 a.axillaris

臂丛神经 plexus brachialis

胸廓内动脉 a.thoracica interna

肋间神经 nervi intercostales

肋间动静脉 a.v.intercostales

腹壁上动静脉 a.v.epigastrica superior

白线 linea alba

腹壁下动静脉 a.v.epigastrica inferior

股动静脉 a.v.femoralis

大隐静脉 vena saphena magna

肋间神经前皮支 ramus cutaneus anterior (n. intercostales)

肋间神经外侧皮支 ramus cutaneus lateralis (n. intercostales)

肋间神经前皮支 ramus cutaneus anterior (n. intercostales)

脐 umbilicus

肋间神经外侧皮支 ramus cutaneus lateralis (n. intercostales)

股外侧皮神经 nervus cutaneus femoris lateralis

精索 funiculus spermaticus

股中间皮神经 n. cutaneus femoris intermedius

(RN22) (KI27) (ST13) (LU2) (LU1) (RN20) (ST15) (SP20) (KI24) (SP19) (SP18) (RN17) (KI22) (ST18) (SP17) (RN14) (KI21) (RN11) (KI18) (SP16) (LR13) (KI16) (ST25) (RN7) (SP14) (KI14) (RN4) (ST28) (KI12) (RN2) (SP12)

Fig. 22 The blood vessels, nerves and points on the anterior aspect of the trunk   35

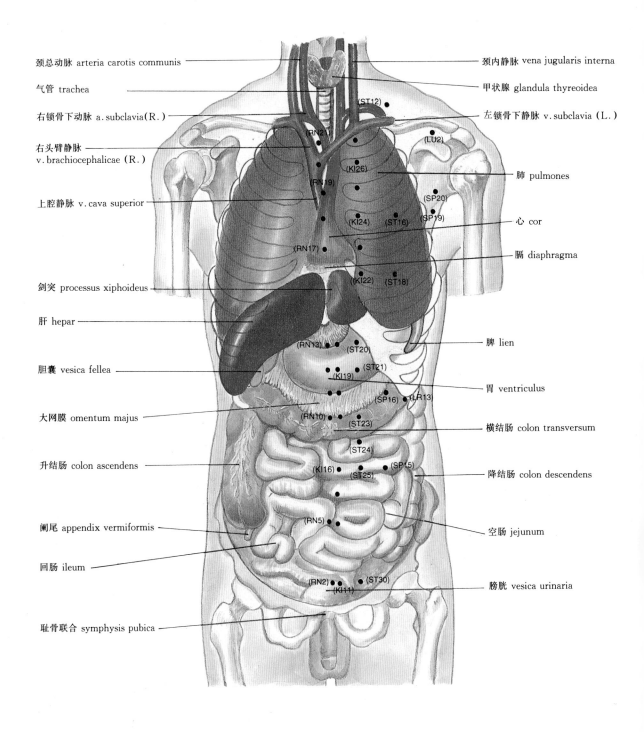

颈总动脉 arteria carotis communis
气管 trachea
右锁骨下动脉 a. subclavia(R.)
右头臂静脉 v. brachiocephalicae (R.)
上腔静脉 v. cava superior
剑突 processus xiphoideus
肝 hepar
胆囊 vesica fellea
大网膜 omentum majus
升结肠 colon ascendens
阑尾 appendix vermiformis
回肠 ileum
耻骨联合 symphysis pubica

颈内静脉 vena jugularis interna
甲状腺 glandula thyreoidea
左锁骨下静脉 v. subclavia (L.)
肺 pulmones
心 cor
膈 diaphragma
脾 lien
胃 ventriculus
横结肠 colon transversum
降结肠 colon descendens
空肠 jejunum
膀胱 vesica urinaria

(ST12)
(RN21)
(LU2)
(KI26)
(RN19)
(SP20)
(KI24) (ST16) (SP19)
(RN17)
(KI22) (ST18)
(RN13) (ST20)
(KI19) (ST21)
(SP16) (LR13)
(RN10) (ST23)
(ST24)
(KI16) (SP15)
(ST25)
(RN5)
(RN2) (ST30)
(KI11)

36

Fig. 23 The organs and points on the anterior aspect of the trunk

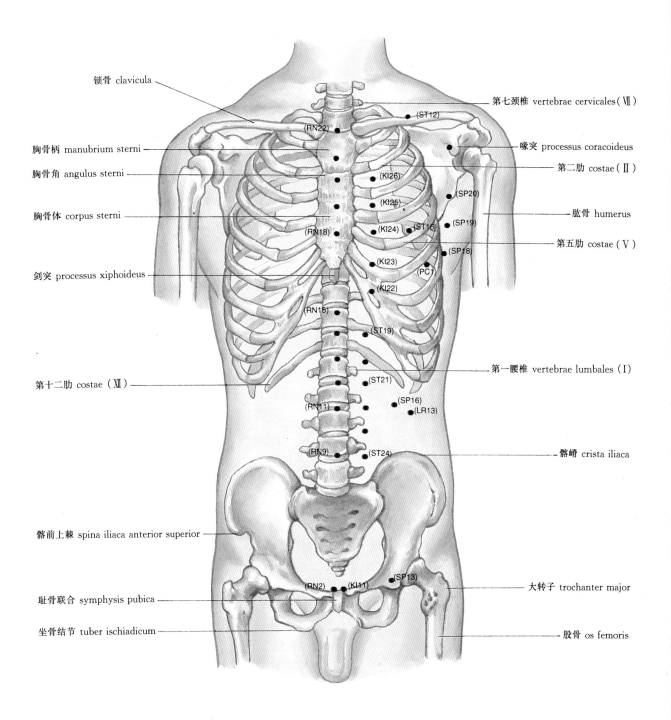

Fig. 24 The skeleton and points on the anterior aspect of the trunk

37

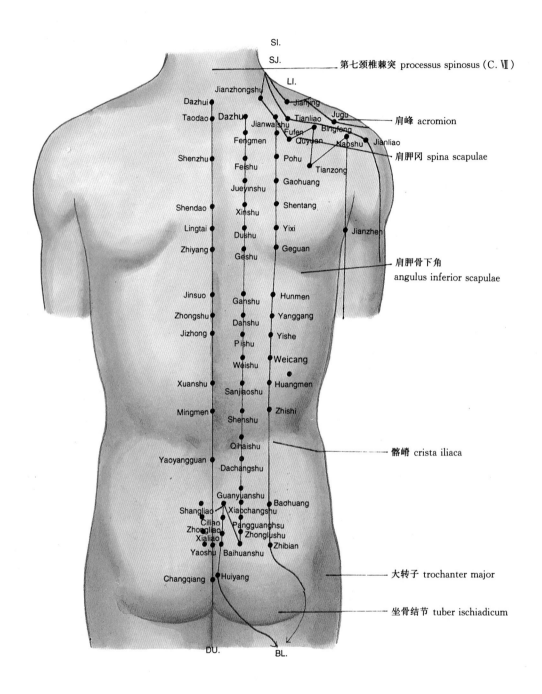

SI.

SJ.

第七颈椎棘突 processus spinosus (C. Ⅶ)

LI.

Jianzhongshu

Dazhui

Taodao   Dazhu

Jianjing   Jugu   肩峰 acromion

Jianwaishu   Tianliao   Bingfeng

Fengmen   Fufen   Jianliao

Quyuan   Naoshu   肩胛冈 spina scapulae

Shenzhu   Pohu

Feishu   Tianzong

Jueyinshu   Gaohuang

Shendao   Xinshu   Shentang

Lingtai   Dushu   Yixi

Zhiyang   Geshu   Geguan

Jianzhen

肩胛骨下角
angulus inferior scapulae

Jinsuo   Ganshu   Hunmen

Zhongshu   Dashu   Yanggang

Jizhong   Pishu   Yishe

Weishu   Weicang

Xuanshu   Sanjiaoshu   Huangmen

Mingmen   Shenshu   Zhishi

Qihaishu

Yaoyangguan   Dachangshu   髂嵴 crista iliaca

Guanyuanshu   Baohuang

Shangliao   Xiaochangshu
Ciliao   Pangguanghsu
Zhongliao   Zhonglushu
Xialiao
Yaoshu   Baihuanshu   Zhibian

大转子 trochanter major

Changqiang   Huiyang

坐骨结节 tuber ischiadicum

DU.   BL.

38   **Fig. 25 The skin and points on the posterior aspect of the trunk**

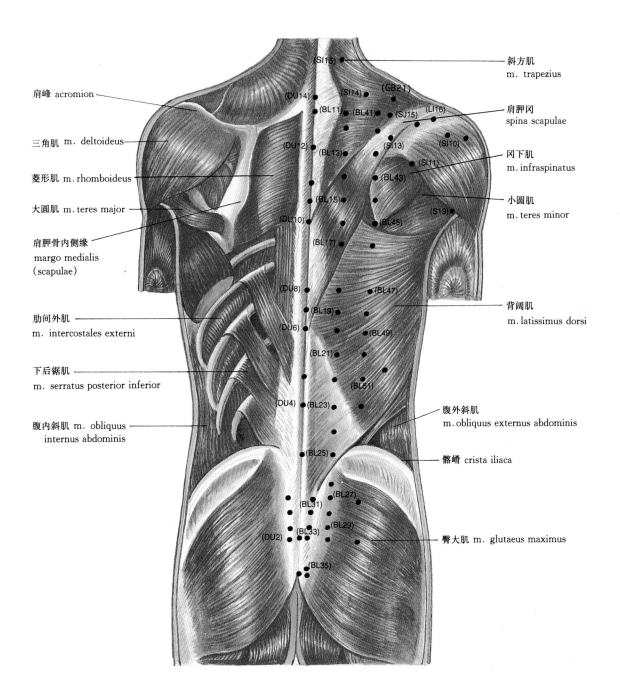

Fig. 26 The muscles and points on the posterior aspect of the trunk

39

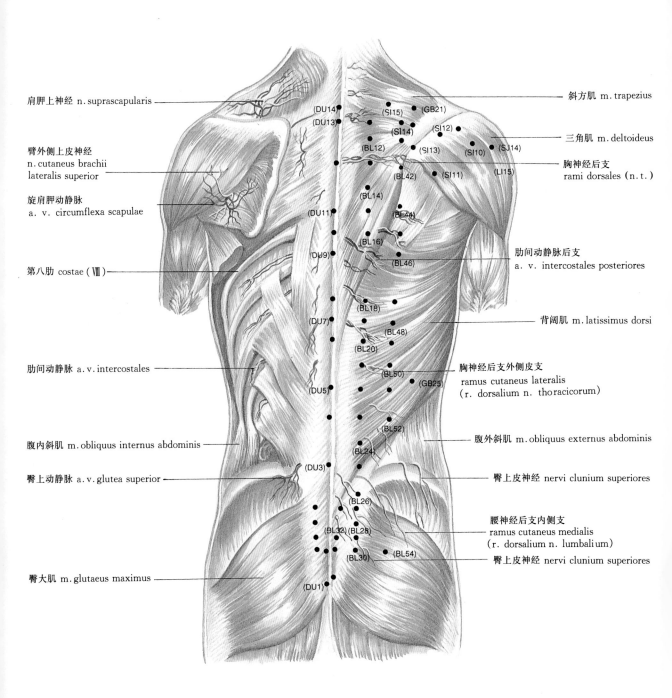

肩胛上神经 n.suprascapularis

臂外侧上皮神经
n.cutaneus brachii
lateralis superior

旋肩胛动静脉
a. v. circumflexa scapulae

第八肋 costae (Ⅷ)

肋间动静脉 a.v.intercostales

腹内斜肌 m.obliquus internus abdominis

臀上动静脉 a.v.glutea superior

臀大肌 m.glutaeus maximus

斜方肌 m.trapezius

三角肌 m.deltoideus

胸神经后支
rami dorsales (n.t.)

肋间动静脉后支
a. v. intercostales posteriores

背阔肌 m.latissimus dorsi

胸神经后支外侧皮支
ramus cutaneus lateralis
(r. dorsalium n. thoracicorum)

腹外斜肌 m.obliquus externus abdominis

臀上皮神经 nervi clunium superiores

腰神经后支内侧支
ramus cutaneus medialis
(r. dorsalium n. lumbalium)

臀上皮神经 nervi clunium superiores

(DU14) (SI15) (GB21)
(DU13) (SI14) (SI12)
(BL12) (SI13) (SI10) (SJ14)
(BL42) (SI11) (LI15)
(BL14)
(DU11) (BL44)
(BL16)
(DU9) (BL46)
(BL18)
(DU7) (BL48)
(BL20)
(BL50) (GB25)
(DU5)
(BL52)
(BL24)
(DU3)
(BL26)
(BL32)(BL28)
(BL30) (BL54)
(DU1)

Fig. 27 The blood vessels, nerves and points on the posterior aspect of the trunk

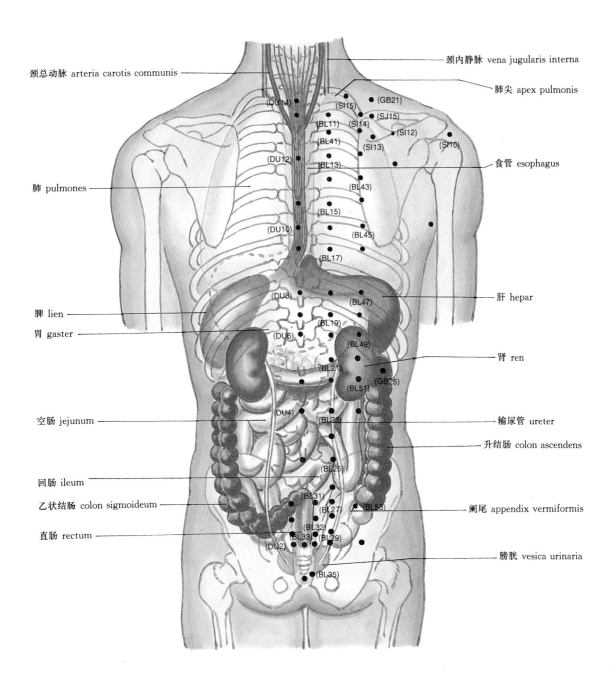

颈总动脉 arteria carotis communis

颈内静脉 vena jugularis interna

肺尖 apex pulmonis

(DU14)

(SI15)　(GB21)

(SJ15)

(BL11)　(SI14)

(BL41)　　(SI12)

(SI13)　　(SI10)

(DU12)

(BL13)

食管 esophagus

肺 pulmones

(BL43)

(BL15)

(DU10)

(BL45)

(BL17)

(DU8)　　(BL47)

肝 hepar

脾 lien

(BL19)

胃 gaster

(DU6)

(BL49)

肾 ren

(BL21)

(BL51)　(GB25)

(DU4)

(BL23)

输尿管 ureter

空肠 jejunum

升结肠 colon ascendens

(BL25)

回肠 ileum

(BL31)

乙状结肠 colon sigmoideum

(BL27)　(BL53)

阑尾 appendix vermiformis

(BL32)

直肠 rectum

(BL33)　(BL29)

(DU2)

膀胱 vesica urinaria

(BL35)

Fig. 28 The organs and points on the posterior aspect of the trunk　　41

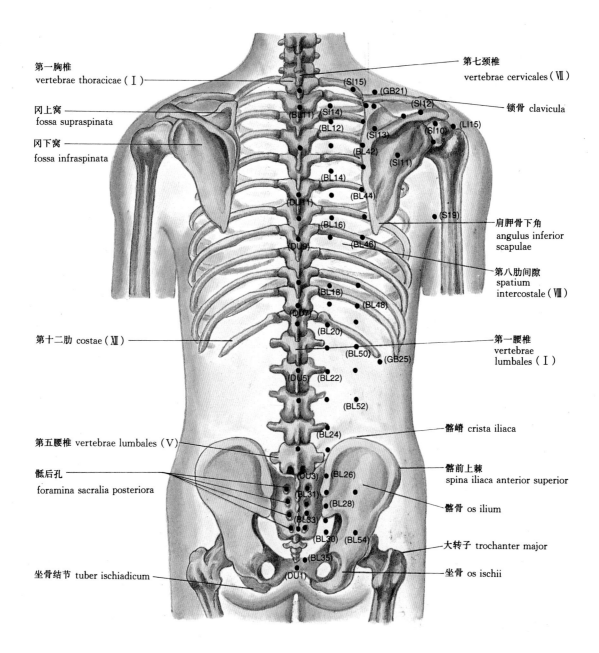

第一胸椎
vertebrae thoracicae（Ⅰ）

冈上窝
fossa supraspinata

冈下窝
fossa infraspinata

第十二肋 costae（ⅩⅡ）

第五腰椎 vertebrae lumbales（Ⅴ）

骶后孔
foramina sacralia posteriora

坐骨结节 tuber ischiadicum

第七颈椎
vertebrae cervicales（Ⅶ）

锁骨 clavicula

肩胛骨下角
angulus inferior
scapulae

第八肋间隙
spatium
intercostale（Ⅷ）

第一腰椎
vertebrae
lumbales（Ⅰ）

髂嵴 crista iliaca

髂前上棘
spina iliaca anterior superior

髂骨 os ilium

大转子 trochanter major

坐骨 os ischii

(SI15)
(GB21)
(SI12)
(BL11) (SI14)
(BL12)
(SI13)
(SI10)
(LI15)
(BL42)
(SI11)
(BL14)
(BL44)
(DU11)
(S19)
(BL16)
(DU9)
(BL46)
(BL18)
(BL48)
(DU7)
(BL20)
(BL50)
(GB25)
(DU5) (BL22)
(BL52)
(BL24)
(DU3) (BL26)
(BL31)
(BL28)
(BL33)
(BL30) (BL54)
(BL35)
(DU1)

Fig. 29 The skeleton and points on the posterior aspect of the trunk

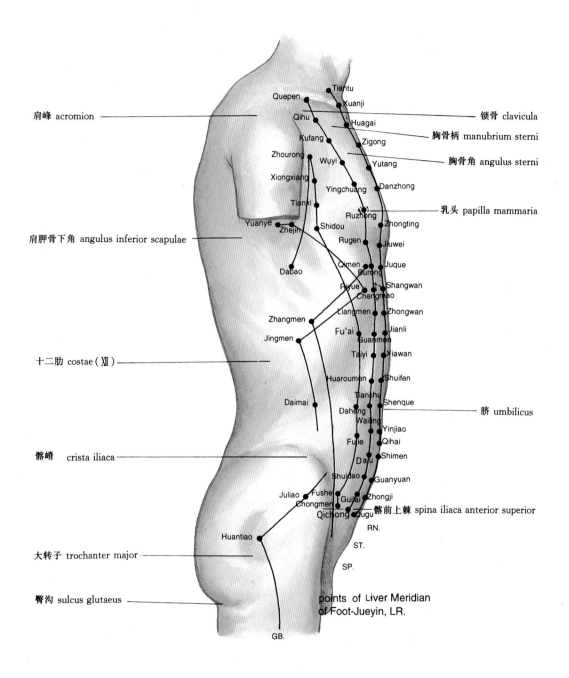

肩峰 acromion

锁骨 clavicula

胸骨柄 manubrium sterni

胸骨角 angulus sterni

乳头 papilla mammaria

肩胛骨下角 angulus inferior scapulae

十二肋 costae (XII)

脐 umbilicus

髂嵴 crista iliaca

髂前上棘 spina iliaca anterior superior

大转子 trochanter major

臀沟 sulcus glutaeus

Tiantu
Quepen
Xuanji
Qihu
Huagai
Kufang
Zigong
Zhourong
Wuyi
Yutang
Xiongxiang
Yingchuang
Danzhong
Tianxi
Ruzhong
Yuanye
Shidou
Zhongting
Zhejin
Rugen
Jiuwei
Dabao
Qimen
Juque
Burong
Fuyue
Shangwan
Chengman
Liangmen
Zhongwan
Zhangmen
Fu'ai
Jianli
Jingmen
Guanmen
Taiyi
Xiawan
Huaroumen
Shuifen
Tianshu
Daimai
Shenque
Daheng
Wailing
Yinjiao
Fujie
Qihai
Daju
Shimen
Shuidao
Guanyuan
Juliao
Fushe
Zhongji
Chongmen
Guilai
Qichong Qugu

RN.
ST.
SP.

points of Liver Meridian
of Foot-Jueyin, LR.

Huantiao

GB.

Fig. 30 The skin and points on the right aspect of the trunk

43

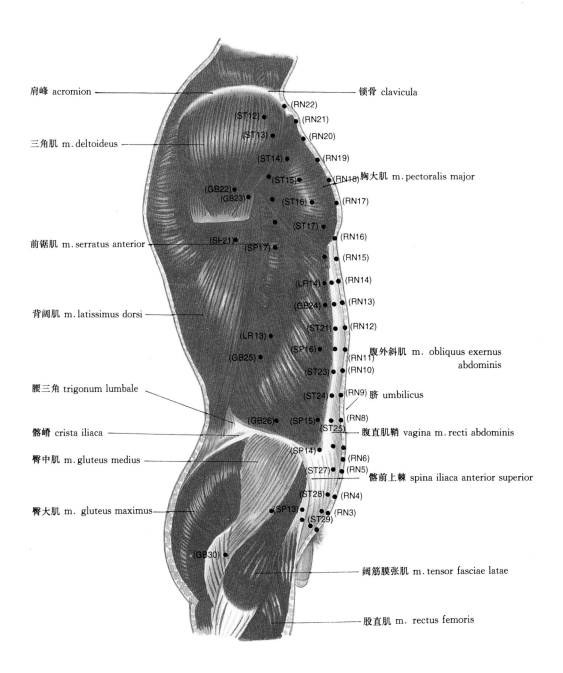

肩峰 acromion

三角肌 m.deltoideus

前锯肌 m.serratus anterior

背阔肌 m.latissimus dorsi

腰三角 trigonum lumbale

髂嵴 crista iliaca

臀中肌 m.gluteus medius

臀大肌 m.gluteus maximus

锁骨 clavicula

(ST12)
(ST13)
(ST14)
(ST15)
(GB22)
(GB23)
(ST16)
(ST17)
(ST21)
(SP17)
(LR14)
(GB24)
(ST21)
(LR13)
(SP16)
(GB25)
(ST23)
(ST24)
(GB26)
(SP15)
(ST25)
(SP14)
(ST27)
(ST28)
(SP13)
(ST29)
(GB30)

(RN22)
(RN21)
(RN20)
(RN19)
(RN18)
(RN17)
(RN16)
(RN15)
(RN14)
(RN13)
(RN12)
(RN11)
(RN10)
(RN9)
(RN8)
(RN6)
(RN5)
(RN4)
(RN3)

胸大肌 m.pectoralis major

腹外斜肌 m.obliquus exernus abdominis

脐 umbilicus

腹直肌鞘 vagina m.recti abdominis

髂前上棘 spina iliaca anterior superior

阔筋膜张肌 m.tensor fasciae latae

股直肌 m.rectus femoris

Fig. 31 The muscles and points on the right aspect of the trunk

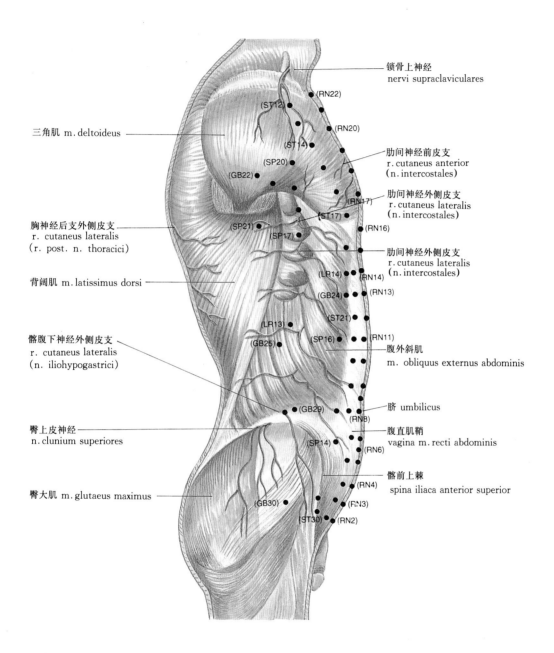

锁骨上神经
nervi supraclaviculares

(RN22)

(ST12)

(RN20)

三角肌 m. deltoideus

(ST14)

(SP20)

肋间神经前皮支
r. cutaneus anterior
(n. intercostales)

(GB22)

(RN17)

肋间神经外侧皮支
r. cutaneus lateralis
(n. intercostales)

(ST17)

(RN16)

胸神经后支外侧皮支
r. cutaneus lateralis
(r. post. n. thoracici)

(SP21)

(SP17)

肋间神经外侧皮支
r. cutaneus lateralis
(n. intercostales)

(LR14)

(RN14)

背阔肌 m. latissimus dorsi

(GB24)

(RN13)

(ST21)

(LR13)

(SP16)

(RN11)

髂腹下神经外侧皮支
r. cutaneus lateralis
(n. iliohypogastrici)

(GB25)

腹外斜肌
m. obliquus externus abdominis

(GB29)

脐 umbilicus

(RN8)

臀上皮神经
n. clunium superiores

腹直肌鞘
vagina m. recti abdominis

(SP14)

(RN6)

髂前上棘
spina iliaca anterior superior

(RN4)

臀大肌 m. gluteaus maximus

(GB30)

(RN3)

(ST30)

(RN2)

Fig. 32 The blood vessels, nerves and points on the right aspect of the trunk   45

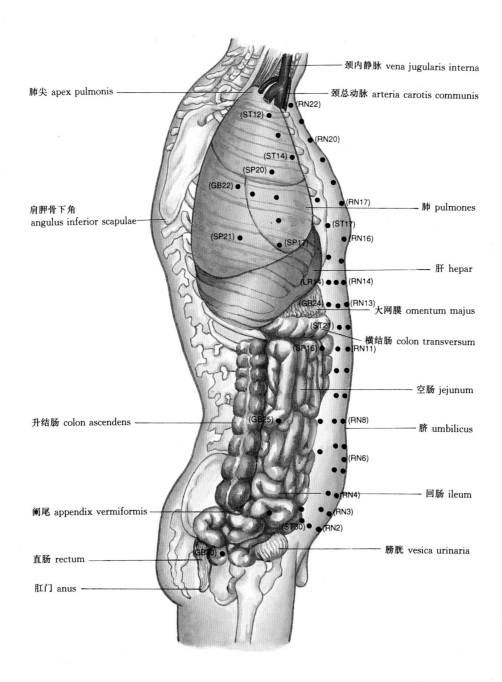

颈内静脉 vena jugularis interna

肺尖 apex pulmonis

颈总动脉 arteria carotis communis

(RN22)

(ST12)

(RN20)

(ST14)

(SP20)

(GB22)

(RN17) 肺 pulmones

(ST17)

(SP21)

(SP17)

(RN16)

肝 hepar

(LR14) (RN14)

(GB24) (RN13)

大网膜 omentum majus

肩胛骨下角
angulus inferior scapulae

(ST21)

横结肠 colon transversum

(SP16) (RN11)

空肠 jejunum

升结肠 colon ascendens

(GB25)

(RN8)

脐 umbilicus

(RN6)

回肠 ileum

(RN4)

阑尾 appendix vermiformis

(RN3)

(ST30) (RN2)

直肠 rectum

(GB30)

膀胱 vesica urinaria

肛门 anus

46   **Fig. 33 The organs and points on the right aspect of the trunk**

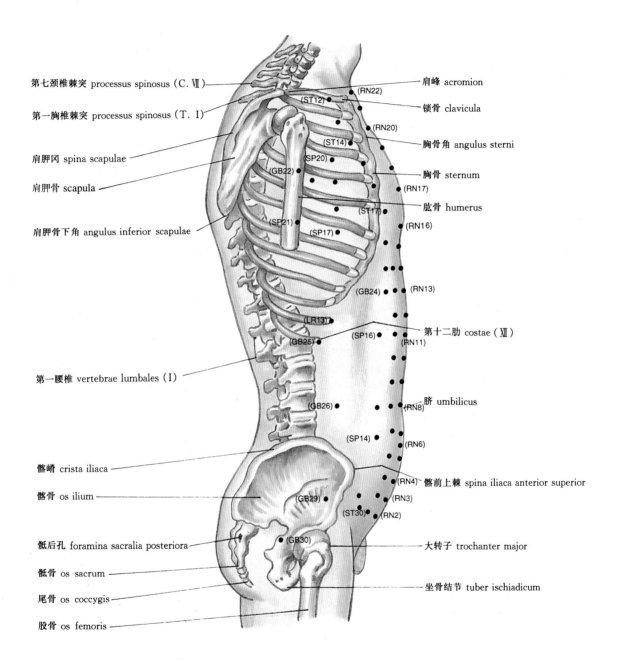

第七颈椎棘突 processus spinosus（C.Ⅶ）

第一胸椎棘突 processus spinosus（T.Ⅰ）

肩胛冈 spina scapulae

肩胛骨 scapula

肩胛骨下角 angulus inferior scapulae

第一腰椎 vertebrae lumbales（Ⅰ）

髂嵴 crista iliaca

髂骨 os ilium

骶后孔 foramina sacralia posteriora

骶骨 os sacrum

尾骨 os coccygis

股骨 os femoris

肩峰 acromion

锁骨 clavicula

胸骨角 angulus sterni

胸骨 sternum

肱骨 humerus

第十二肋 costae（Ⅻ）

脐 umbilicus

髂前上棘 spina iliaca anterior superior

大转子 trochanter major

坐骨结节 tuber ischiadicum

(RN22)
(ST12)
(RN20)
(ST14)
(SP20)
(GB22)
(RN17)
(ST17)
(SP21)
(RN16)
(SP17)
(GB24)
(RN13)
(LR13)
(SP16)
(GB25)
(RN11)
(GB26)
(RN8)
(SP14)
(RN6)
(RN4)
(GB29)
(RN3)
(ST30)
(RN2)
(GB30)

Fig. 34 The skeleton and points on the right aspect of the trunk

47

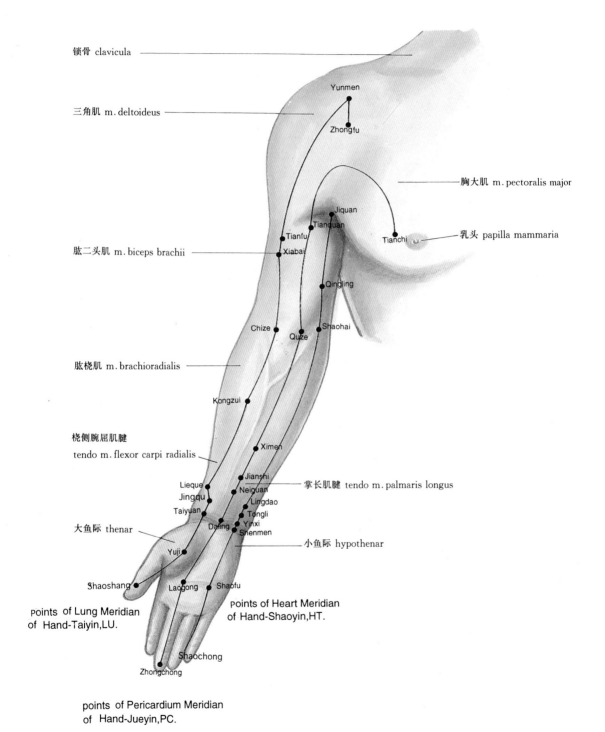

锁骨 clavicula

三角肌 m. deltoideus

胸大肌 m. pectoralis major

乳头 papilla mammaria

肱二头肌 m. biceps brachii

肱桡肌 m. brachioradialis

桡侧腕屈肌腱
tendo m. flexor carpi radialis

掌长肌腱 tendo m. palmaris longus

大鱼际 thenar

小鱼际 hypothenar

Yunmen

Zhongfu

Jiquan

Tianquan

Tianfu

Xiabai

Qingling

Tianchi

Chize

Quze

Shaohai

Kongzui

Ximen

Jianshi

Lieque

Neiguan

Jingqu

Lingdao

Taiyuan

Tongli

Daling

Yinxi

Shenmen

Yuji

Shaoshang

Laogong

Shaofu

points of Lung Meridian
of Hand-Taiyin, LU.

points of Heart Meridian
of Hand-Shaoyin, HT.

Shaochong

Zhongchong

points of Pericardium Meridian
of Hand-Jueyin, PC.

48   **Fig. 35 The skin and points on the anterior aspect of the right upper limb**

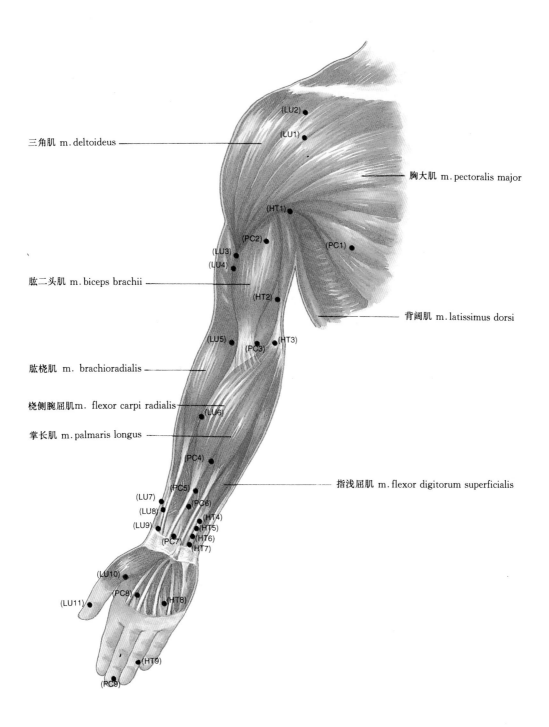

三角肌 m. deltoideus

胸大肌 m. pectoralis major

(LU2)

(LU1)

(HT1)

(PC2)

(PC1)

(LU3)

(LU4)

肱二头肌 m. biceps brachii

(HT2)

背阔肌 m. latissimus dorsi

(LU5)

(HT3)

(PC3)

肱桡肌 m. brachioradialis

桡侧腕屈肌m. flexor carpi radialis

(LU6)

掌长肌 m. palmaris longus

(PC4)

指浅屈肌 m. flexor digitorum superficialis

(PC5)

(LU7)

(PC6)

(LU8)

(HT4)

(LU9)

(HT5)

(PC7)

(HT6)

(HT7)

(LU10)

(PC8)

(HT8)

(LU11)

(HT9)

(PC9)

Fig. 36 The muscles and points on the anterior aspect of the right upper limb   49

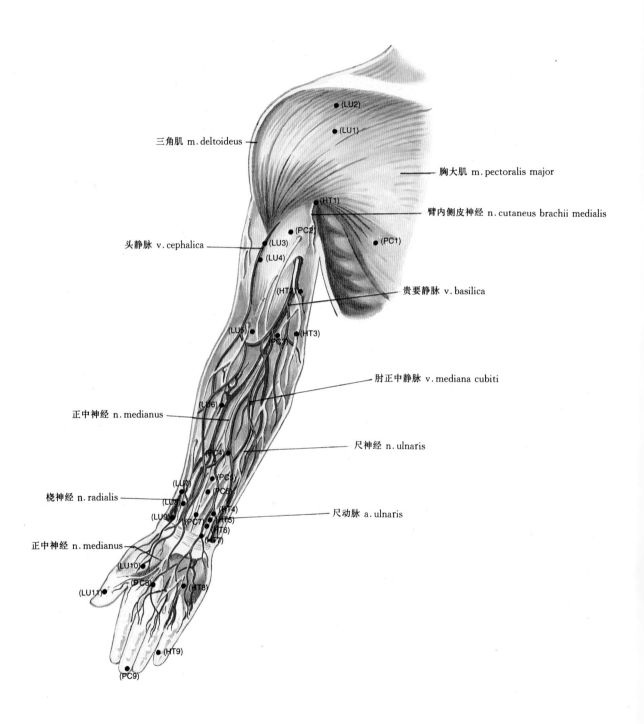

三角肌 m. deltoideus

胸大肌 m. pectoralis major

臂内侧皮神经 n. cutaneus brachii medialis

头静脉 v. cephalica

贵要静脉 v. basilica

肘正中静脉 v. mediana cubiti

正中神经 n. medianus

尺神经 n. ulnaris

桡神经 n. radialis

尺动脉 a. ulnaris

正中神经 n. medianus

(LU2)
(LU1)
(HT1)
(PC2)
(LU3)
(PC1)
(LU4)
(HT2)
(LU5)
(PC3)
(HT3)
(LU6)
(PC4)
(PC5)
(LU7)
(PC6)
(LU8)
(HT4)
(LU9)
(HT5)
(PC7)
(HT6)
(HT7)
(LU10)
(PC8)
(HT8)
(LU11)
(HT9)
(PC9)

50   **Fig. 37 The blood vessels, nerves and points on the anterior aspect of the right upper limb**

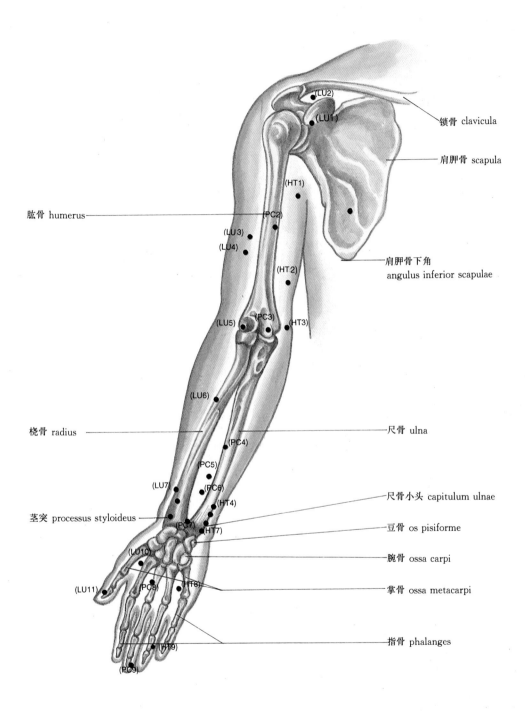

锁骨 clavicula

肩胛骨 scapula

肩胛骨下角
angulus inferior scapulae

肱骨 humerus

桡骨 radius

尺骨 ulna

尺骨小头 capitulum ulnae

豆骨 os pisiforme

腕骨 ossa carpi

掌骨 ossa metacarpi

茎突 processus styloideus

指骨 phalanges

Fig. 38 The skeleton and points on the anterior aspect of the right upper limb   51

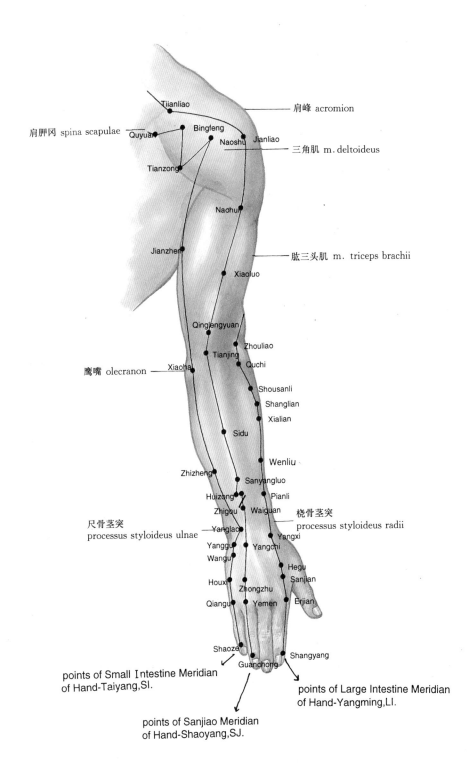

Tiianliao

肩峰 acromion

肩胛冈 spina scapulae

Quyuan

Bingfeng

Naoshu

Jianliao

三角肌 m. deltoideus

Tianzong

Naohui

Jianzhen

肱三头肌 m. triceps brachii

Xiaoluo

Qinglengyuan

Zhouliao

Tianjing

Quchi

鹰嘴 olecranon — Xiaohai

Shousanli

Shanglian

Xialian

Sidu

Wenliu

Zhizheng

Sanyangluo

Huizong

Pianli

Zhigou

Waiguan

尺骨茎突
processus styloideus ulnae

桡骨茎突
processus styloideus radii

Yanglao

Yangxi

Yanggu

Yangchi

Wangu

Hegu

Houxi

Sanjian

Zhongzhu

Qiangu

Yemen

Erjian

Shaoze

Shangyang

points of Small Intestine Meridian
of Hand-Taiyang,SI.

Guanchong

points of Large Intestine Meridian
of Hand-Yangming,LI.

points of Sanjiao Meridian
of Hand-Shaoyang,SJ.

52   **Fig. 39 The skin and points on the posterior aspect of the right upper limb**

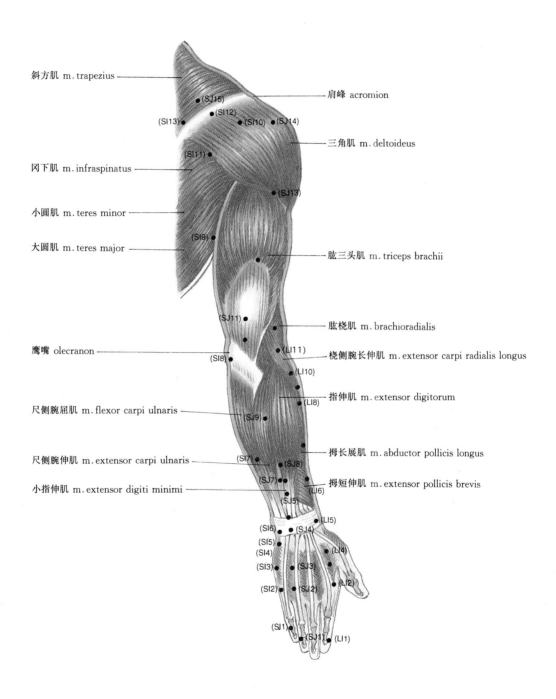

斜方肌 m. trapezius —

肩峰 acromion

(SJ15)
(SI12)
(SI13)
(SI10) (SJ14)

三角肌 m. deltoideus

(SI11)

冈下肌 m. infraspinatus —

(SJ13)

小圆肌 m. teres minor —

大圆肌 m. teres major —

(SI9)

肱三头肌 m. triceps brachii

(SJ11)

肱桡肌 m. brachioradialis

(LI11)

鹰嘴 olecranon —

桡侧腕长伸肌 m. extensor carpi radialis longus

(SI8)

(LI10)

指伸肌 m. extensor digitorum

(LI8)

尺侧腕屈肌 m. flexor carpi ulnaris —

(SJ9)

拇长展肌 m. abductor pollicis longus

尺侧腕伸肌 m. extensor carpi ulnaris —

(SI7)
(SJ8)

拇短伸肌 m. extensor pollicis brevis

(SJ7)

小指伸肌 m. extensor digiti minimi —

(LI6)
(SJ5)

(SI6) (SJ4) (LI5)

(SI5)

(SI4) (LI4)

(SI3) (SJ3)

(SI2) (SJ2) (LI2)

(SI1) (SJ1) (LI1)

Fig. 40 The muscles and points on the posterior aspect of the right upper limb

53

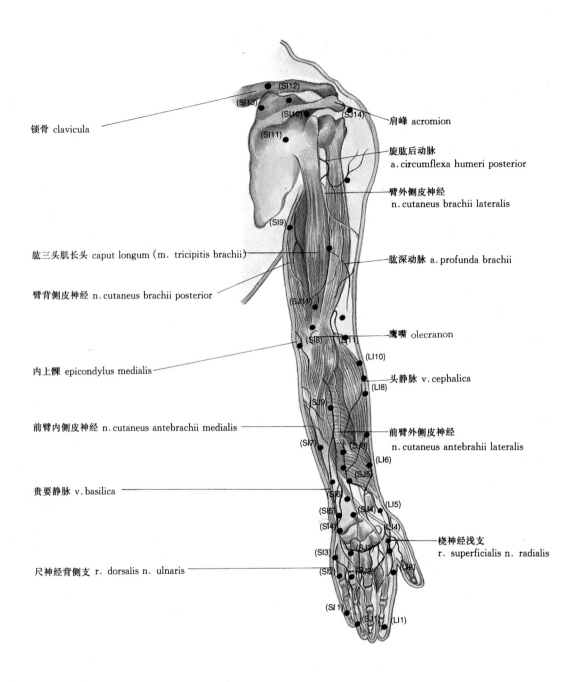

锁骨 clavicula

(SI12)
(SI13)
(SI10)
(SJ14)
(SI11)
肩峰 acromion

旋肱后动脉
a. circumflexa humeri posterior

臂外侧皮神经
n. cutaneus brachii lateralis

(SI9)

肱三头肌长头 caput longum (m. tricipitis brachii)

肱深动脉 a. profunda brachii

臂背侧皮神经 n. cutaneus brachii posterior

(SJ11)

鹰嘴 olecranon

(SI8) (LI11)

(LI10)

内上髁 epicondylus medialis

头静脉 v. cephalica

(LI8)

(SJ9)

前臂内侧皮神经 n. cutaneus antebrachii medialis

前臂外侧皮神经
n. cutaneus antebrahii lateralis

(SI7)

(SJ8)

(LI6)

(SJ5)

贵要静脉 v. basilica

(SI6)

(SJ4) (LI5)

(SI5)

(SI4)

(LI4)

桡神经浅支
r. superficialis n. radialis

(SI3)

(SJ3)

尺神经背侧支 r. dorsalis n. ulnaris

(SI2)

(SJ2)

(LI2)

(SI 1)

(SJ1) (LI1)

54   **Fig. 41 The blood vessels, nerves and points on the posterior aspect of the right upper limb**

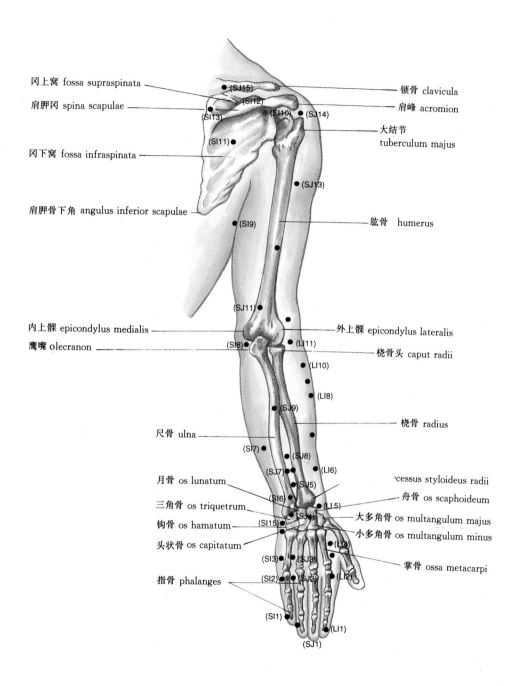

冈上窝 fossa supraspinata

肩胛冈 spina scapulae

冈下窝 fossa infraspinata

肩胛骨下角 angulus inferior scapulae

内上髁 epicondylus medialis

鹰嘴 olecranon

尺骨 ulna

月骨 os lunatum

三角骨 os triquetrum

钩骨 os hamatum

头状骨 os capitatum

指骨 phalanges

锁骨 clavicula

肩峰 acromion

大结节 tuberculum majus

肱骨 humerus

外上髁 epicondylus lateralis

桡骨头 caput radii

桡骨 radius

'cessus styloideus radii

舟骨 os scaphoideum

大多角骨 os multangulum majus

小多角骨 os multangulum minus

掌骨 ossa metacarpi

(SJ15)
(SI12)
(SI13)
(SI10) (SJ14)
(SI11)
(SJ13)
(SI9)
(SJ11)
(SI8) (LI11)
(LI10)
(LI8)
(SJ9)
(SI7)
(SJ8)
(SJ7) (LI6)
(SJ5)
(SI6) (LI5)
(SI15) (SJ4)
(SI3) (SJ3)
(LI4)
(SI2) (SJ2) (LI2)
(SI1)
(LI1)
(SJ1)

Fig. 42 The skeleton and points on the posterior aspect of the right upper limb   55

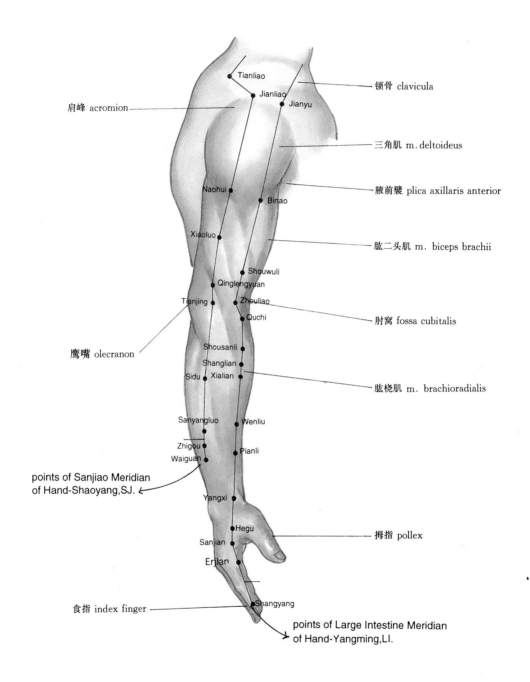

Tianliao

Jianliao

Jianyu

锁骨 clavicula

肩峰 acromion

三角肌 m. deltoideus

Naohui

Binao

腋前襞 plica axillaris anterior

Xiaoluo

肱二头肌 m. biceps brachii

Shouwuli

Qinglengyuan

Zhouliao

Tianjing

Quchi

肘窝 fossa cubitalis

Shousanli

Shanglian

鹰嘴 olecranon

Sidu

Xialian

肱桡肌 m. brachioradialis

Sanyangluo

Wenliu

Zhigou

Pianli

Waiguan

points of Sanjiao Meridian
of Hand-Shaoyang,SJ.

Yangxi

Hegu

拇指 pollex

Sanjian

Erjian

食指 index finger

Shangyang

points of Large Intestine Meridian
of Hand-Yangming,LI.

56   **Fig. 43 The skin and points on the lateral aspect of the right upper limb**

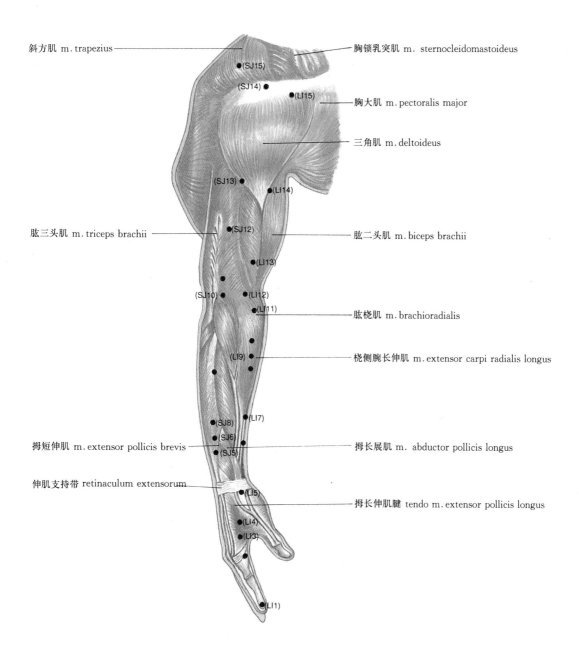

斜方肌 m.trapezius

胸锁乳突肌 m.sternocleidomastoideus

● (SJ15)

(SJ14) ●
● (LI15)

胸大肌 m.pectoralis major

三角肌 m.deltoideus

(SJ13) ●
● (LI14)

肱三头肌 m.triceps brachii

● (SJ12)

肱二头肌 m.biceps brachii

● (LI13)

(SJ10) ●
● (LI12)
● (LI11)

肱桡肌 m.brachioradialis

(LI9) ●

桡侧腕长伸肌 m.extensor carpi radialis longus

● (LI7)

● (SJ8)
● (SJ6)
● (SJ5)

拇短伸肌 m.extensor pollicis brevis

拇长展肌 m.abductor pollicis longus

伸肌支持带 retinaculum extensorum

● (LI5)

拇长伸肌腱 tendo m.extensor pollicis longus

● (LI4)
● (LI3)

● (LI1)

Fig. 44 The muscles and points on the lateral aspect of the right upper limb

57

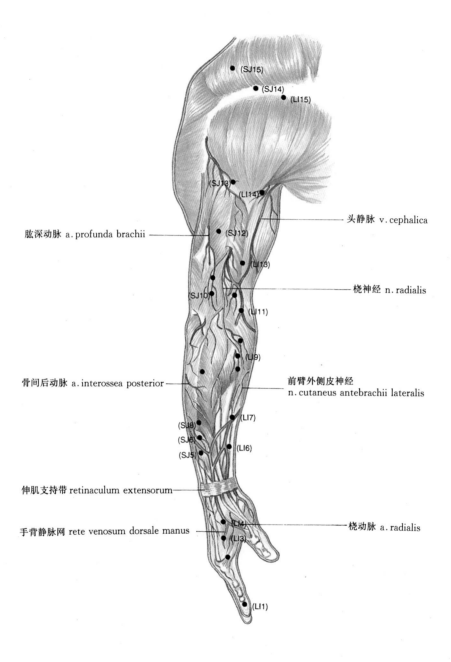

头静脉 v. cephalica

肱深动脉 a. profunda brachii

桡神经 n. radialis

骨间后动脉 a. interossea posterior

前臂外侧皮神经
n. cutaneus antebrachii lateralis

伸肌支持带 retinaculum extensorum

桡动脉 a. radialis

手背静脉网 rete venosum dorsale manus

(SJ15)
(SJ14)
(LI15)
(SJ13)
(LI14)
(SJ12)
(LI13)
(SJ10)
(LI11)
(LI9)
(LI7)
(SJ8)
(SJ6)
(LI6)
(SJ5)
(LI4)
(LI3)
(LI1)

Fig. 45 The blood vessels, nerves and points on the lateral aspect of the right upper limb

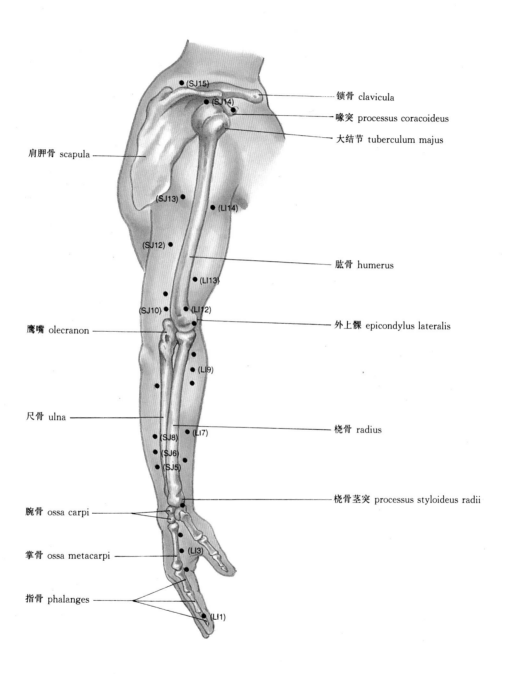

● (SJ15)

● (SJ14)

锁骨 clavicula

喙突 processus coracoideus

大结节 tuberculum majus

肩胛骨 scapula

(SJ13) ●

● (LI14)

(SJ12) ●

肱骨 humerus

● (LI13)

(SJ10) ●   ● (LI12)

鹰嘴 olecranon

外上髁 epicondylus lateralis

● (LI9)

尺骨 ulna

桡骨 radius

● (LI7)

● (SJ8)

● (SJ6)

● (SJ5)

桡骨茎突 processus styloideus radii

腕骨 ossa carpi

掌骨 ossa metacarpi

● (LI3)

指骨 phalanges

● (LI1)

Fig. 46 The skeleton and points on the lateral aspect of the right upper limb   59

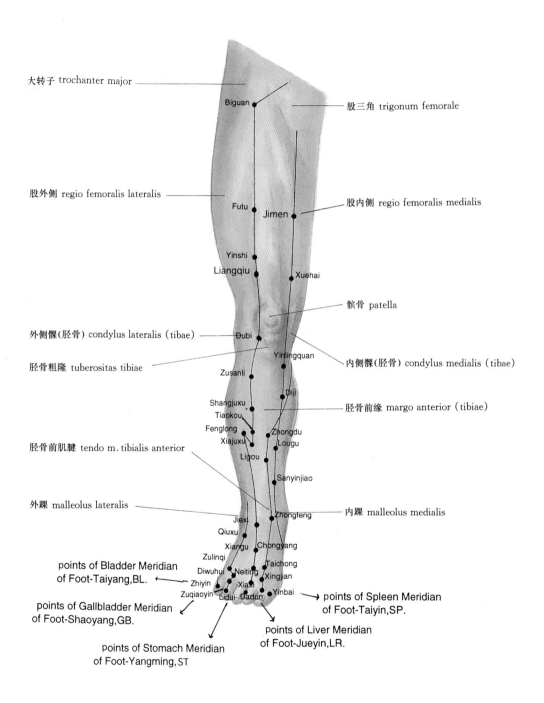

大转子 trochanter major

Biguan

股三角 trigonum femorale

股外侧 regio femoralis lateralis

Futu

Jimen

股内侧 regio femoralis medialis

Yinshi

Liangqiu

Xuehai

髌骨 patella

外侧髁(胫骨) condylus lateralis (tibae)

Dubi

Yinlingquan

内侧髁(胫骨) condylus medialis (tibae)

胫骨粗隆 tuberositas tibiae

Zusanli

Diji

Shangjuxu

胫骨前缘 margo anterior (tibiae)

Tiaokou

Fenglong

Zhongdu

Xiajuxu

Lougu

胫骨前肌腱 tendo m. tibialis anterior

Ligou

Sanyinjiao

外踝 malleolus lateralis

Zhongfeng

内踝 malleolus medialis

Jiexi

Qiuxu

Xiangu

Chongyang

Zulinqi

Taichong

points of Bladder Meridian
of Foot-Taiyang, BL.

Diwuhui

Neiting

Xingjian

Zhiyin

Xiaxi

Yinbai

points of Spleen Meridian
of Foot-Taiyin, SP.

Zuqiaoyin

Lidui

Dadun

points of Gallbladder Meridian
of Foot-Shaoyang, GB.

points of Liver Meridian
of Foot-Jueyin, LR.

points of Stomach Meridian
of Foot-Yangming, ST

Fig. 47 The skin and points on the anterior aspect of the right lower limb

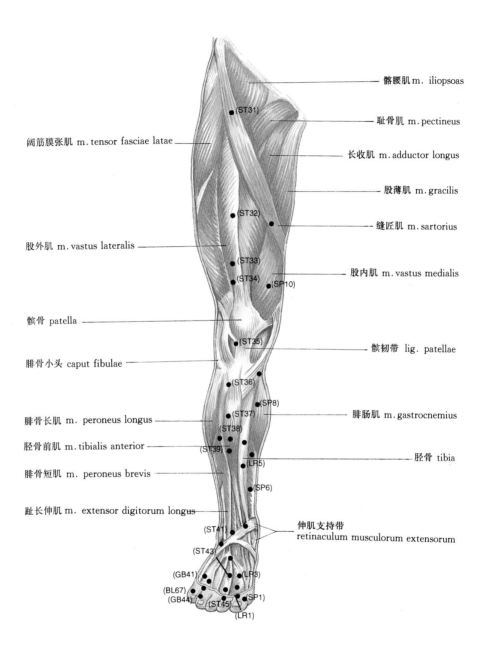

髂腰肌 m. iliopsoas

耻骨肌 m. pectineus

长收肌 m. adductor longus

股薄肌 m. gracilis

缝匠肌 m. sartorius

股内肌 m. vastus medialis

髌韧带 lig. patellae

腓肠肌 m. gastrocnemius

胫骨 tibia

伸肌支持带
retinaculum musculorum extensorum

阔筋膜张肌 m. tensor fasciae latae

股外肌 m. vastus lateralis

髌骨 patella

腓骨小头 caput fibulae

腓骨长肌 m. peroneus longus

胫骨前肌 m. tibialis anterior

腓骨短肌 m. peroneus brevis

趾长伸肌 m. extensor digitorum longus

(ST31)
(ST32)
(ST33)
(ST34)
(SP10)
(ST35)
(ST36)
(SP8)
(ST37)
(ST38)
(ST39)
(LR5)
(SP6)
(ST41)
(ST43)
(GB41)
(LR3)
(BL67)
(GB44)
(ST45)
(SP1)
(LR1)

Fig. 48 The muscles and points on the anterior aspect of the right lower limb

61

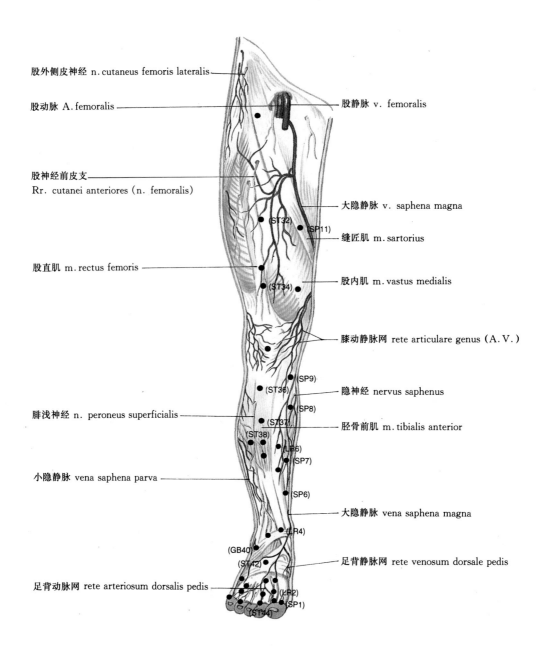

股外侧皮神经 n. cutaneus femoris lateralis

股动脉 A. femoralis

股神经前皮支
Rr. cutanei anteriores（n. femoralis）

股直肌 m. rectus femoris

腓浅神经 n. peroneus superficialis

小隐静脉 vena saphena parva

足背动脉网 rete arteriosum dorsalis pedis

股静脉 v. femoralis

大隐静脉 v. saphena magna

缝匠肌 m. sartorius

股内肌 m. vastus medialis

膝动静脉网 rete articulare genus（A. V.）

隐神经 nervus saphenus

胫骨前肌 m. tibialis anterior

大隐静脉 vena saphena magna

足背静脉网 rete venosum dorsale pedis

(ST32)
(SP11)
(ST34)
(SP9)
(ST36)
(SP8)
(ST37)
(ST38)
(LR6)
(SP7)
(SP6)
(LR4)
(GB40)
(ST42)
(LR2)
(SP1)
(ST44)

62　　**Fig. 49 The blood vessels, nerves and points on the anterior aspect of the right lower limb**

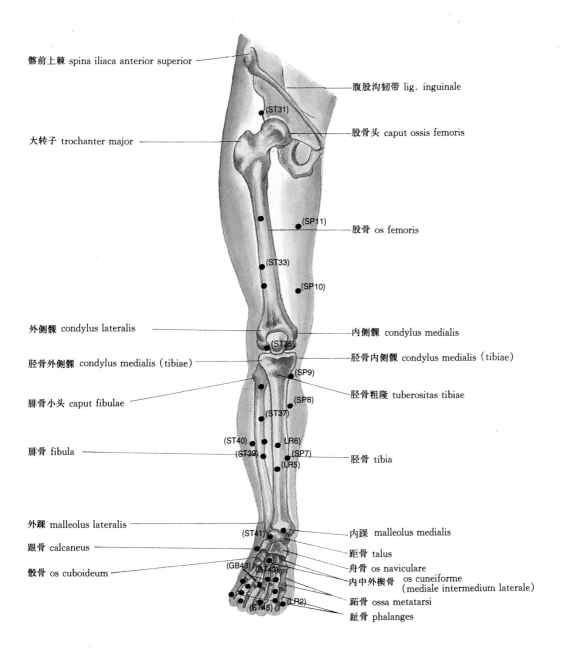

髂前上棘 spina iliaca anterior superior

腹股沟韧带 lig. inguinale

(ST31)

股骨头 caput ossis femoris

大转子 trochanter major

(SP11)

股骨 os femoris

(ST33)

(SP10)

外侧髁 condylus lateralis

内侧髁 condylus medialis

胫骨外侧髁 condylus medialis（tibiae）

(ST35)

胫骨内侧髁 condylus medialis（tibiae）

(SP9)

胫骨粗隆 tuberositas tibiae

腓骨小头 caput fibulae

(SP8)

(ST37)

腓骨 fibula

(ST40)　LR6

(ST39)　(SP7)

(LR5)

胫骨 tibia

外踝 malleolus lateralis

内踝 malleolus medialis

跟骨 calcaneus

(ST41)

距骨 talus

骰骨 os cuboideum

(GB43)　(ST43)

舟骨 os naviculare

内中外楔骨 os cuneiforme
（mediale intermedium laterale）

距骨 ossa metatarsi

(ST45)　LR2

趾骨 phalanges

Fig. 50 The skeleton and points on the anterior aspect of the right lower limb　　63

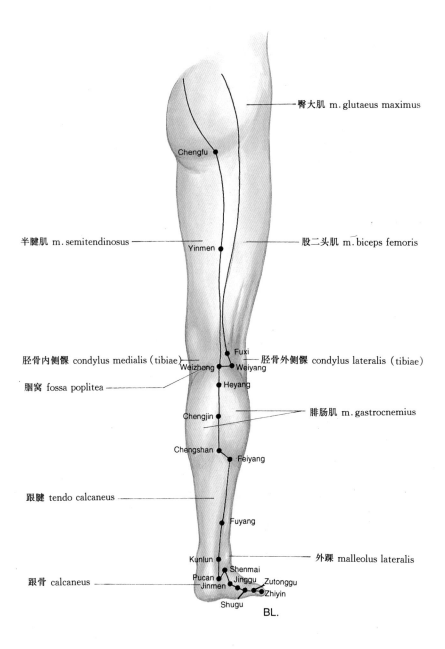

臀大肌 m. glutaeus maximus

Chengfu

半腱肌 m. semitendinosus

Yinmen

股二头肌 m. biceps femoris

Fuxi

胫骨内侧髁 condylus medialis (tibiae)

Weizhong

Weiyang

胫骨外侧髁 condylus lateralis (tibiae)

腘窝 fossa poplitea

Heyang

Chengjin

腓肠肌 m. gastrocnemius

Chengshan

Feiyang

跟腱 tendo calcaneus

Fuyang

Kunlun

外踝 malleolus lateralis

Shenmai

Pucan

Jinggu

Zutonggu

跟骨 calcaneus

Jinmen

Zhiyin

Shugu

BL.

Fig. 51 The skin and points on the posterior aspect of the right lower limb

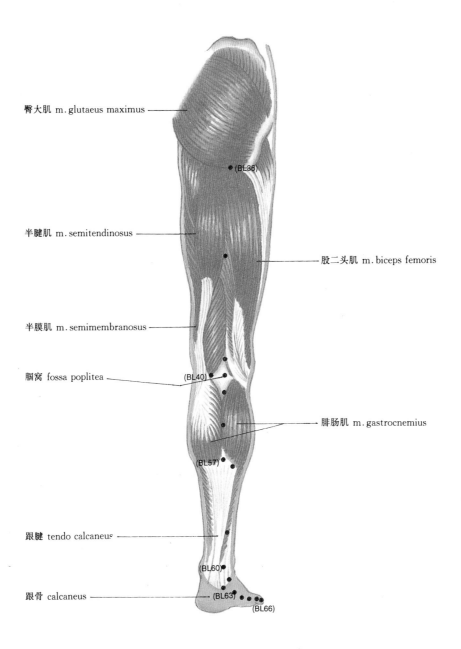

臀大肌 m. glutaeus maximus

(BL36)

半腱肌 m. semitendinosus

股二头肌 m. biceps femoris

半膜肌 m. semimembranosus

腘窝 fossa poplitea

(BL40)

腓肠肌 m. gastrocnemius

(BL57)

跟腱 tendo calcaneus

(BL60)

跟骨 calcaneus

(BL63)

(BL66)

Fig. 52 The muscles and points on the posterior aspect of the right lower limb

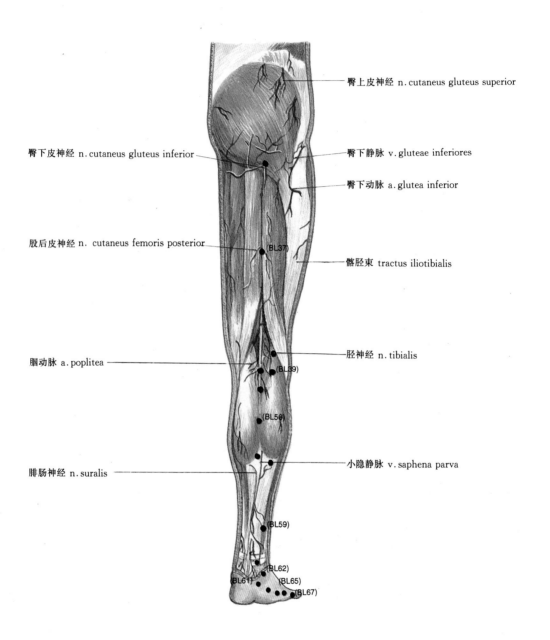

臀上皮神经 n. cutaneus gluteus superior

臀下皮神经 n. cutaneus gluteus inferior

臀下静脉 v. gluteae inferiores

臀下动脉 a. glutea inferior

股后皮神经 n. cutaneus femoris posterior

(BL37)

髂胫束 tractus iliotibialis

胫神经 n. tibialis

腘动脉 a. poplitea

(BL39)

(BL56)

小隐静脉 v. saphena parva

腓肠神经 n. suralis

(BL59)

(BL62)

(BL61)   (BL65)

(BL67)

66   **Fig. 53 The blood vessels, nerves and points on the posterior aspect of the right lower limb**

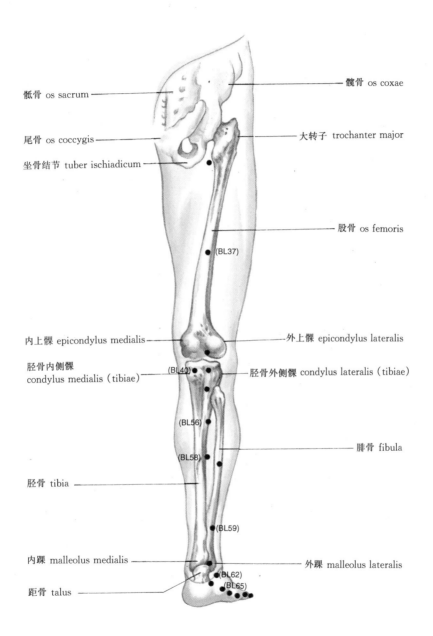

骶骨 os sacrum

尾骨 os coccygis

坐骨结节 tuber ischiadicum

内上髁 epicondylus medialis

胫骨内侧髁
condylus medialis（tibiae）

胫骨 tibia

内踝 malleolus medialis

距骨 talus

髋骨 os coxae

大转子 trochanter major

股骨 os femoris

外上髁 epicondylus lateralis

胫骨外侧髁 condylus lateralis（tibiae）

腓骨 fibula

外踝 malleolus lateralis

(BL37)

(BL40)

(BL56)

(BL58)

(BL59)

(BL62)

(BL65)

Fig. 54 The skeleton and points on the posterior aspect of the right lower limb   67

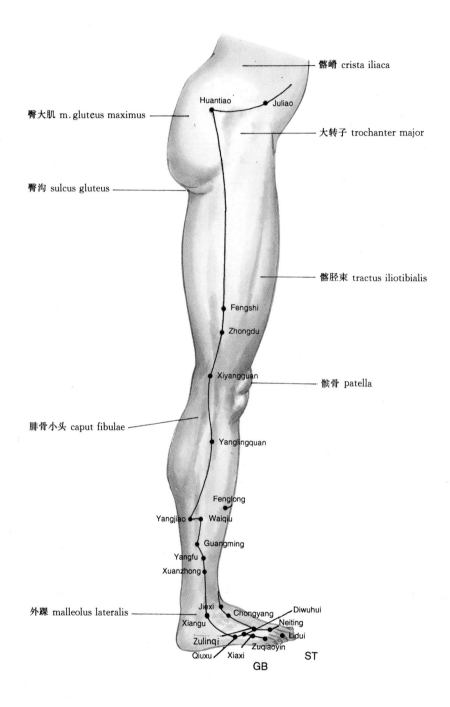

髂嵴 crista iliaca

臀大肌 m. gluteus maximus

Huantiao

Juliao

大转子 trochanter major

臀沟 sulcus gluteus

髂胫束 tractus iliotibialis

Fengshi

Zhongdu

Xiyangguan

髌骨 patella

腓骨小头 caput fibulae

Yanglingquan

Fenglong

Yangjiao

Waiqiu

Guangming

Yangfu

Xuanzhong

外踝 malleolus lateralis

Jiexi

Chongyang

Diwuhui

Xiangu

Neiting

Lidui

Zulinqi

Zuqiaoyin

Qiuxu

Xiaxi

ST

GB

Fig. 55 The skin and points on the lateral aspect of the right lower limb

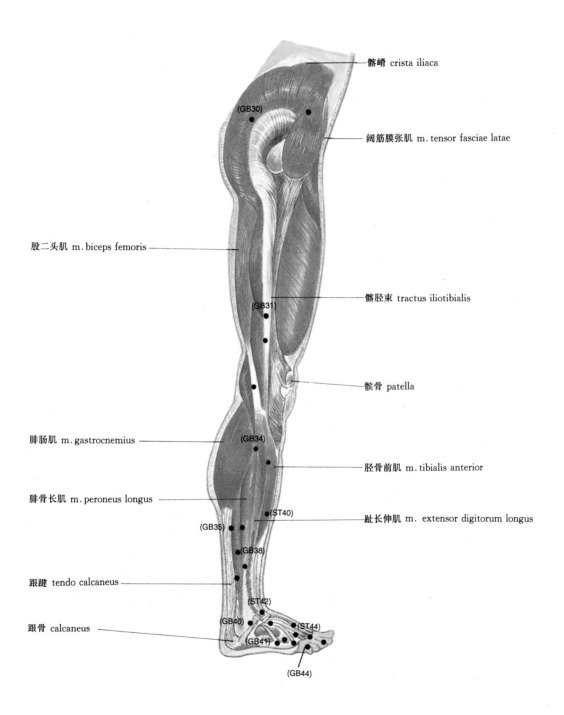

髂嵴 crista iliaca

(GB30)

阔筋膜张肌 m. tensor fasciae latae

股二头肌 m. biceps femoris

髂胫束 tractus iliotibialis

(GB31)

髌骨 patella

腓肠肌 m. gastrocnemius

(GB34)

胫骨前肌 m. tibialis anterior

腓骨长肌 m. peroneus longus

(ST40)

趾长伸肌 m. extensor digitorum longus

(GB35)

(GB38)

跟腱 tendo calcaneus

(ST42)

跟骨 calcaneus

(GB40)

(ST44)

(GB41)

(GB44)

Fig. 56 The muscles and points on the lateral aspect of the right lower limb

69

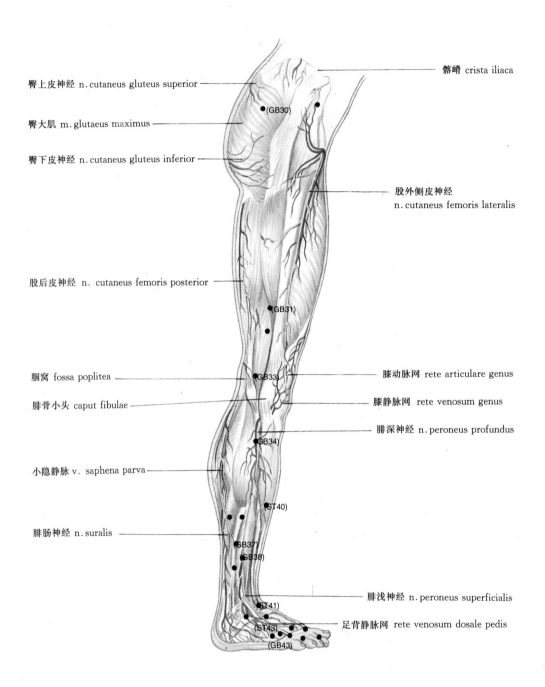

臀上皮神经 n. cutaneus gluteus superior

臀大肌 m. glutaeus maximus

臀下皮神经 n. cutaneus gluteus inferior

股后皮神经 n. cutaneus femoris posterior

腘窝 fossa poplitea

腓骨小头 caput fibulae

小隐静脉 v. saphena parva

腓肠神经 n. suralis

髂嵴 crista iliaca

(GB30)

股外侧皮神经
n. cutaneus femoris lateralis

(GB31)

(GB33)　膝动脉网 rete articulare genus

膝静脉网 rete venosum genus

腓深神经 n. peroneus profundus

(GB34)

(ST40)

(GB37)

(GB38)

腓浅神经 n. peroneus superficialis

(ST41)

(ST43)　足背静脉网 rete venosum dosale pedis

(GB43)

70　**Fig. 57 The blood vessels, nerves and points on the lateral aspect of the right lower limb**

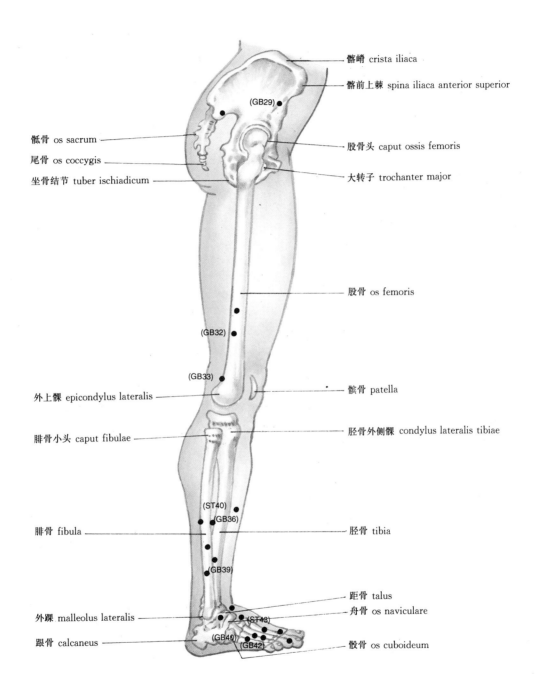

髂嵴 crista iliaca

髂前上棘 spina iliaca anterior superior

(GB29)

骶骨 os sacrum

尾骨 os coccygis

坐骨结节 tuber ischiadicum

股骨头 caput ossis femoris

大转子 trochanter major

股骨 os femoris

(GB32)

(GB33)

髌骨 patella

外上髁 epicondylus lateralis

胫骨外侧髁 condylus lateralis tibiae

腓骨小头 caput fibulae

(ST40)

(GB36)

腓骨 fibula

胫骨 tibia

(GB39)

距骨 talus

舟骨 os naviculare

外踝 malleolus lateralis

(ST43)

跟骨 calcaneus

(GB40)

(GB42)

骰骨 os cuboideum

Fig. 58 The skeleton and points on the lateral aspect of the right lower limb   71

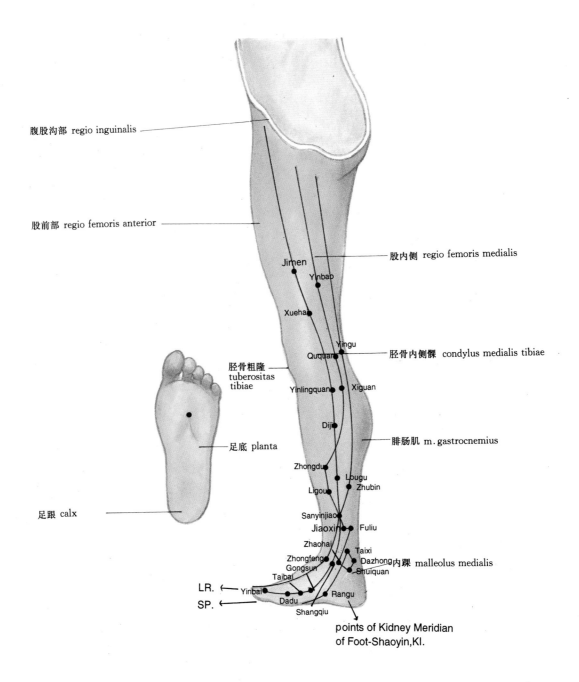

腹股沟部 regio inguinalis

股前部 regio femoris anterior

股内侧 regio femoris medialis

Jimen

Yinbao

Xuehai

Yingu

Ququan

胫骨内侧髁 condylus medialis tibiae

胫骨粗隆 tuberositas tibiae

Yinlingquan

Xiguan

Diji

足底 planta

腓肠肌 m. gastrocnemius

Zhongdu

Lougu

Zhubin

Ligou

足跟 calx

Sanyinjiao

Jiaoxin

Fuliu

Zhaohai

Taixi

Zhongfeng

Dazhong 内踝 malleolus medialis

Gongsun

Shuiquan

Taibai

LR.

Yinbai

SP.

Dadu

Rangu

Shangqiu

points of Kidney Meridian
of Foot-Shaoyin, KI.

72   **Fig. 59 The skin and points on the medial aspect of the right lower limb**

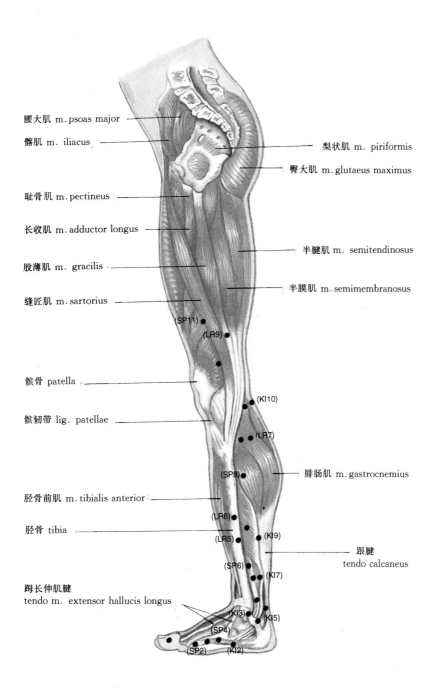

腰大肌 m. psoas major

髂肌 m. iliacus

耻骨肌 m. pectineus

长收肌 m. adductor longus

股薄肌 m. gracilis

缝匠肌 m. sartorius

髌骨 patella

髌韧带 lig. patellae

胫骨前肌 m. tibialis anterior

胫骨 tibia

踇长伸肌腱
tendo m. extensor hallucis longus

梨状肌 m. piriformis

臀大肌 m. gluteus maximus

半腱肌 m. semitendinosus

半膜肌 m. semimembranosus

腓肠肌 m. gastrocnemius

跟腱
tendo calcaneus

(SP11)
(LR9)
(KI10)
(LR7)
(SP8)
(LR6)
(LR5) (KI9)
(SP6)
(KI7)
(KI3)
(KI5)
(SP4)
(SP2) (KI2)

Fig. 60 The muscles and points on the medial aspect of the right lower limb

73

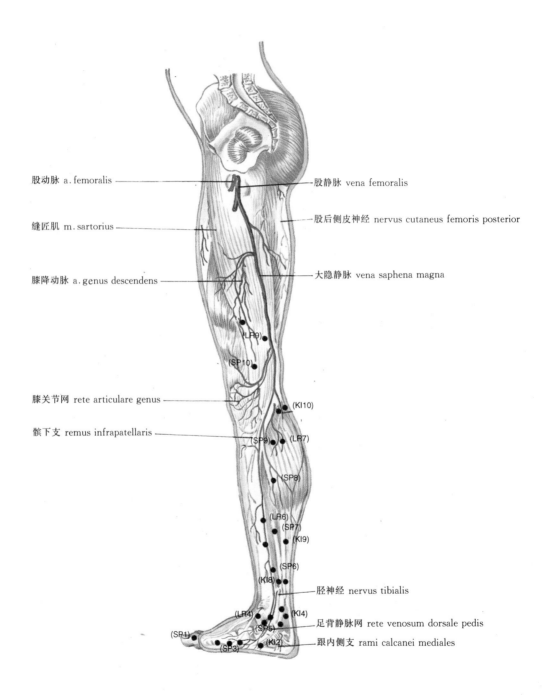

股动脉 a. femoralis

缝匠肌 m. sartorius

膝降动脉 a. genus descendens

膝关节网 rete articulare genus

髌下支 remus infrapatellaris

股静脉 vena femoralis

股后侧皮神经 nervus cutaneus femoris posterior

大隐静脉 vena saphena magna

(LR9)

(SP10)

(KI10)

(SP9)   (LR7)

(SP8)

(LR6)
(SP7)
(KI9)

(SP6)

(KI8)

胫神经 nervus tibialis

(LR4)   (KI4)

足背静脉网 rete venosum dorsale pedis

(SP5)

跟内侧支 rami calcanei mediales

(SP1)

(KI2)

(SP3)

74   **Fig. 61 The blood vessels, nerves and points on the medial aspect of the right lower limb**

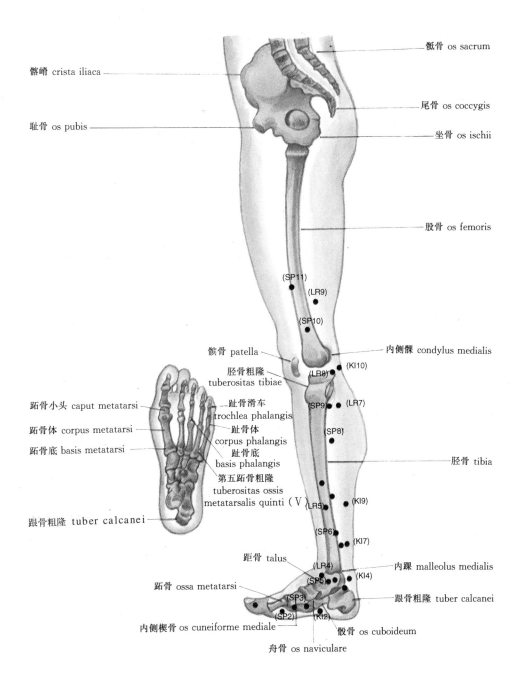

髂嵴 crista iliaca

耻骨 os pubis

骶骨 os sacrum

尾骨 os coccygis

坐骨 os ischii

股骨 os femoris

(SP11)

(LR9)

(SP10)

髌骨 patella

内侧髁 condylus medialis

胫骨粗隆
tuberositas tibiae

(KI10)

(LR8)

趾骨滑车
trochlea phalangis

(SP9)   (LR7)

跖骨小头 caput metatarsi

趾骨体
corpus phalangis

(SP8)

跖骨体 corpus metatarsi

趾骨底
basis phalangis

跖骨底 basis metatarsi

第五跖骨粗隆
tuberositas ossis
metatarsalis quinti（Ⅴ）

胫骨 tibia

跟骨粗隆 tuber calcanei

(LR5)   (KI9)

(SP6)

(KI7)

距骨 talus

(LR4)

内踝 malleolus medialis

(SP5)   (KI4)

跖骨 ossa metatarsi

(SP3)

跟骨粗隆 tuber calcanei

(SP2)   (KI2)

内侧楔骨 os cuneiforme mediale

骰骨 os cuboideum

舟骨 os naviculare

Fig. 62 The skeleton and points on the medial aspect of the right lower limb   75

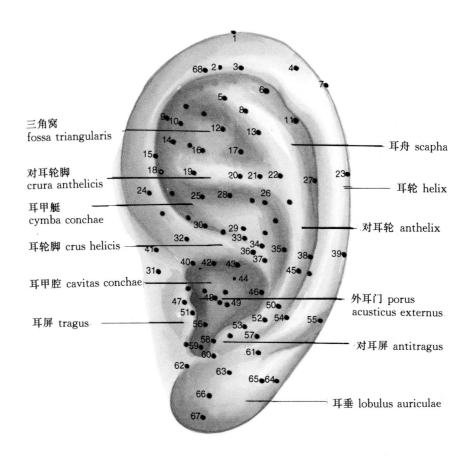

三角窝
fossa triangularis

对耳轮脚
crura anthelicis

耳甲艇
cymba conchae

耳轮脚 crus helicis

耳甲腔 cavitas conchae

耳屏 tragus

耳舟 scapha

耳轮 helix

对耳轮 anthelix

外耳门 porus
acusticus externus

对耳屏 antitragus

耳垂 lobulus auriculae

1 (HX6,7i) 2 (AH 1) 3 (AH 2) 4 (HX 8) 5 (AH 3) 6 (SF 1) 7 (HX 9) 8 (AH 3)
9 (HX 5) 10 (TF 2) 11 (SF 2) 12 (TF 4) 13 (AH 6) 14 (TF 3) 15 (HX 4) 16 (AH 7)
17 (TF 2) 18 (AH6a) 19 (AH 6) 20 (CO 10) 21 (AH 8) 22 (AH 9) 23 (HX 10)
24 (AX 3) 25 (CO 9) 26 (CO 11) 27 (SF 3) 28 (CO9,10i) 29 (CO 6) 30 (CO 7)
31 (TG1u) 32 (HX 2) 33 (CO 6,7i) 34 (CO 5) 35 (CO 12) 36 (HX 1) 37 (CO 4)
38 (SF4) 39 (HX 11) 40 (CO 1) 41 (TG1p) 42 (CO 2) 43 (CO 3) 44 (CO 14)
45 (AH11) 46 (CO 13) 47 (TG1,2i) 48 (CO 16) 49 (CO 15) 50 (SF 6) 51 (TG2p)
52 (AT 2) 53 (AT 1) 54 (AH 13) 55 (HX 12) 56 (CO 17) 57 (AT 3) 58 (AT 4)
59 (CO 18) 60 (LO 2) 61 (LO 3) 62 (LO 1) 63 (LO5,6i) 64 (HX 13) 65 (LO 6)
66 (LO 5) 67 (LO 8) 68 (TF1)

Fig. 63 (1) The skin and points on the anterior aspect of the auricle

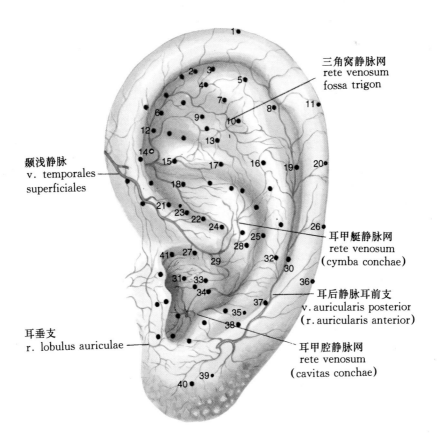

三角窝静脉网
rete venosum
fossa trigon

颞浅静脉
v. temporales
superficiales

耳甲艇静脉网
rete venosum
(cymba conchae)

耳后静脉耳前支
v. auricularis posterior
(r. auricularis anterior)

耳垂支
r. lobulus auriculae

耳甲腔静脉网
rete venosum
(cavitas conchae)

1 (HX6,7i) 2 (AH 1) 3 (AH 2) 4 (AH 3) 5 (SF 1) 6 (TF 2) 7 (AH 4) 8(SF 2) 9 (TF 4)
10 (AH 5) 11 (HX 9) 12 (HX 4) 13 (TF 5) 14 (AH6a) 15 (AH6) 16 (AH 9) 17 (AH7)
18 (CO 9) 19 (SF 3) 20 (HX 10) 21 (CO 7) 22 (CO 6) 23 (CO6,7i) 24 (CO 5)
25 (CO 12) 26 (HX 11) 27 (CO 2) 28 (CO 4) 29 (CO 3) 30 (SF 4) 31 (CO 16)
32 (AH 11) 33 (CO 14) 34 (CO 15) 35 (AH 13) 36 (HX 12) 37 (SF 6) 38 (AT3)
39 (LOS,6i) 40 (LO 5)

Fig. 63 (2) The veins and points on the anterior aspect of the auricle

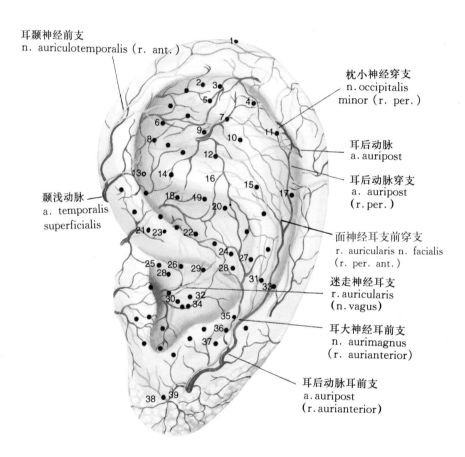

耳颞神经前支
n. auriculotemporalis（r. ant.）

枕小神经穿支
n. occipitalis
minor（r. per.）

耳后动脉
a. auripost

耳后动脉穿支
a. auripost
（r. per.）

颞浅动脉
a. temporalis
superficialis

面神经耳支前穿支
r. auricularis n. facialis
（r. per. ant.）

迷走神经耳支
r. auricularis
（n. vagus）

耳大神经耳前支
n. aurimagnus
（r. aurianterior）

耳后动脉耳前支
a. auripost
（r. aurianterior）

1 (HX6,7i) 2 (AH 1) 3 (AH 2) 4 (SF 1) 5 (AH 3) 6 (TF 2) 7 (AH 4) 8 (HX 4)
9 (TF 4) 10 (AH 5) 11 (SF 2) 12 (TF 5) 13 (AH6a) 14 (AH 6) 15 (AH 9) 16 (AH 7)
17 (SF 3) 18 (CO 9) 19 (CO 10) 20 (CO 11) 21 (CO 7) 22 (CO 6) 23 (CO 6,7i)
24 (CO 5) 25 (CO 1) 26 (CO 2) 27 (CO 12) 28 (CO 3) 29 (CO 4) 30 (CO 16)
31 (AH 11) 32 (CO 14) 33 (SF 4) 34 (CO 15) 35 (SF 6) 36 (AH 13) 37(AH 3)
38 (LO 5) 39 (LO 5,6i)

Fig. 63 (3) The arteries, nerves and points on the anterior aspect of the auricle

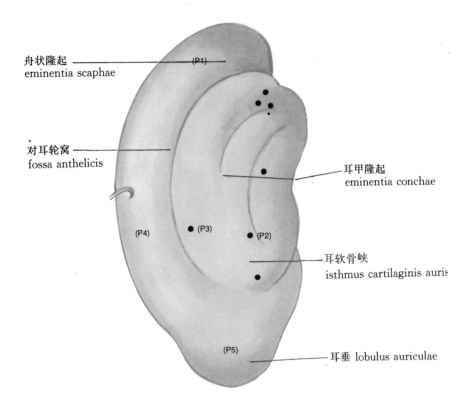

舟状隆起 ——————————— (P1)
eminentia scaphae

对耳轮窝 ———————————
fossa anthelicis

耳甲隆起
eminentia conchae

(P4) ● (P3)   ● (P2)

耳软骨峡
isthmus cartilaginis auris

(P5)

耳垂 lobulus auriculae

Fig. 64 (1) The skin and points on the posterior aspect of the auricle   79

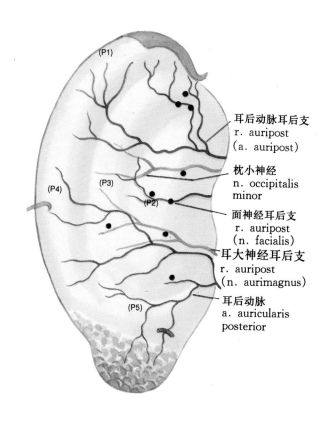

耳后动脉耳后支
r. auripost
(a. auripost)

枕小神经
n. occipitalis
minor

面神经耳后支
r. auripost
(n. facialis)

耳大神经耳后支
r. auripost
(n. aurimagnus)

耳后动脉
a. auricularis
posterior

Fig. 64 (2) The arteries, nerves and points on the posterior aspect of the auricle

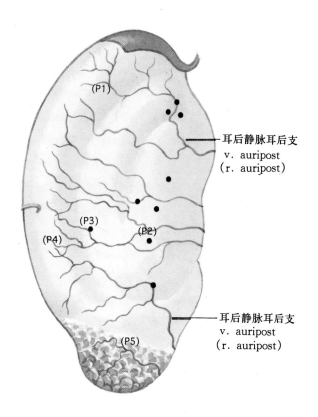

耳后静脉耳后支
v. auripost
（r. auripost）

耳后静脉耳后支
v. auripost
（r. auripost）

Fig. 64 (3) The veins and points on the posterior aspect of the auricle 81

Fig. 65 (1) The distribution of the points on the anterior aspect of the auricle

Helix and points
HX1: ěrzhōng (ear center)
HX2: zhícháng (rectum)
HX3: niàodào (urethra)
HX4: wàishēngzhíqì
 (external genitals)
HX5: gāngmén (anus)
HX6: ěrjiān (ear apex)
HX6, 7i: ěrjiān (ear apex)
HX8: jiéjié (node)
HX9: lúnyí (helix 1)
HX10: lúnèr (helix 2)
HX11: Lúnsān (helix 3)
HX12: lúnsì (helix 4)
HX13: Lúnwǔ (helix 5)
scapha and points
SF1: zhǐ (finger)
SF2: wàn (wrist)
SF1, 2i: fēngxī (wind stream)
SF3: zhǒu (elbow)
SF4, 5: jiān (shoulder)
SF6: suǒgǔ (clavicle)
anthelix and points
AH1: gēn (heel)
AH2: zhǐ (toe)
AH3: huái (ankle)
AH4: xī (knee)
AH5: kuān (hip)
AH6: zuògǔshénjīng
 (sciatic nerve)
AH6a: jiāogǎn (sympathesis)
AH7: tún (gluteus)
AH8: fù (abdomen)
AH9: yāodǐzhuī
 (lumbosacral vertebrae)
AH10: xiōng (chest)
AH11: Xiōngzhuī
 (theracic vertebrae)
AH12: jǐng (neck)
AH13: jǐngzhuī
 (cervical vertebrae)
fossa triangularis and points
TF1: jiǎowōshàng
 (superior triangular fossa)
TF2: Nèishēngzhíqì
 (internal genitals)
TF3: jiǎowōzhōng
 (middle triangular fossa)
TF4: shénmén (shenmen)
TF5: pénqiāng (pelvis)

Iragus and points
TG1: shàngpíng (upper tragus)
TG2: xiàpíng (lower tragus)
TG1u: wàiěi (external ear)
TG1p: píngjiān (apex of tragus)
TG1, 2i: wàibí (external nose)
TG2P: shènshàngxiàn (adrenal gland)
TG3: yānhóu (pharynx and larynx)
TG4: nèibí (internal nose)
antitragus and points
AT1: é (forehead)
AT2: niè (temple)
AT3: zhěn (occiput)
AT4: pízhìxià (subcortex)
conchae auriculae and points
CO1: kǒu (mouth)
CO2: shídào (esophagus)
CO3: bēnmén (cardia)
CO4: wèi (stomach)
CO5: shíèrzhícháng (duodenum)
CO6: xiǎocháng (small intestine)
CO7: dàcháng (large intestine)
CO6, 7i: lánwěi (appendix)
CO8: tīngjiǎo
 (angle of superior concha)
CO9: pángguāng (bladder)
CO10: shèn (kidney)
CO9, 10i: shūniàoguǎn (ureter)
CO11: yídǎn (pancreas and gallbladder)
CO12: gān (liver)
CO13: pí (spleen)
CO14: fèi (lung)
CO15: xīn (heart)
CO16: qìguǎn (trachea)
CO17: sānjiāo (triple energy)
CO18: nèifēnmì (endocrine)
lobulus auriculae and points
LO1: yá (tooth)
LO2: shé (tongue)
LO3: hé (jaw)
LO4: chuíqián (anterior ear lobe)
LO5: yǎn (eye)
LO6: nèiěi (internal ear)
Lo5, 6i: miànjiá (cheek)
LO7, 8, 9: biǎntáotǐ (tonsil)

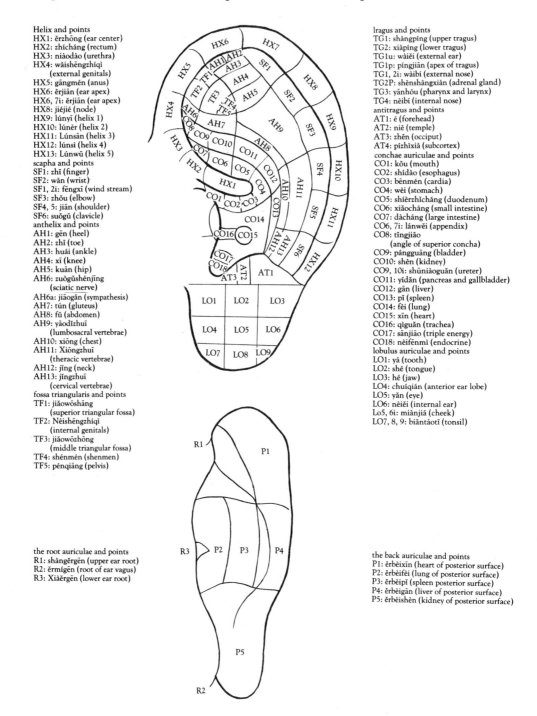

the root auriculae and points
R1: shàngěrgēn (upper ear root)
R2: ěrmígēn (root of ear vagus)
R3: Xiàěrgēn (lower ear root)

the back auriculae and points
P1: ěrbèixīn (heart of posterior surface)
P2: ěrbèifèi (lung of posterior surface)
P3: ěrbèipí (spleen posterior surface)
P4: ěrbèigān (liver of posterior surface)
P5: ěrbèishèn (kidney of posterior surface)

Fig. 65 (2) The distribution of the points on the posterior aspect of the auricle

Appendix 2
The points of the fourteen meridians, the location, the posture of the patient, the direction, angle and depth of insertion of the needle and the indications

1. Face and Eye Region

Point: Yangbai
Meridian: GB 14
Location: On forehead, directly above the pupil, 1 *cun* above eyebrow
Posture: Supine
Angle: Horizontal puncture
Direction: Down
Depth: 6-10 mm
Indications: Frontal headache, dizziness, eye disorders

Point: Jingming
Meridian: BL 1
Location: In depression slightly above the inner canthus
Posture: Spine
Angle: Perpendicular puncture
Direction: Superficial to deep
Depth: 5-10 mm
Indications: Eye disorders (insert slowly, not repeatedly, lifting and thrusting needle)

Point: Cuanzhu
Meridian: BL 2
Location: In depression at medial end of eyebrow, at supraorbital notch
Posture: Supine
Angle: Horizontal
Direction: Above to below
Depth: 6-10 mm
Indications: Eye disorders and headache

Point: Chengqi
Meridian: ST 1
Location: Directly below pupil, between eyeball and infraobital ridge
Posture: Supine
Angle: Perpendicular puncture
Direction: Superficial to deep
Depth: 10-20 mm
Indications: Lacrimation, night blindness, blurred vision

Point: Sibai
Meridian: ST 2
Location: Directly below pupil, in depression of infraobital foramen
Posture: Supine
Angle: Perpendicular puncture
Direction: Superficial to deep
Depth: 6-10 mm
Indications: Headache, facial paralysis, trigeminal neuralgia

Point: Sizhukong
Meridian: SJ 23
Location: In depression on lateral end of eyebrow
Posture: Supine
Angle: Oblique puncture
Direction: Anterior to posterior
Depth: 10-15 mm
Indications: Headache, eye disorders

Point: Tongziliao
Meridian: GB 1
Location: Lateral to outer canthus, on the lateral border of orbit

Posture: Supine
Angle: Oblique puncture
Direction: Laterally
Depth: 6-10 mm
Indications: Headache, eye disorders, facial paralysis

2. Nose and Mouth Region

Point: Suliao
Meridian: DU 25
Location: At center of nasi apex
Posture: Supine
Angle: Oblique puncture
Direction: Upwards
Depth: 5-10 mm
Indications: Pasal disorders, shock, bradycardia

Point: Shuigou
Meridian: DU 26
Location: At junction of upper and middle 1/3 of philtrum
Posture: Supine
Angle: Oblique puncture
Direction: Slightly upwards
Depth: 5-10 mm
Indications: Manic-depression, unconsciousness, infantile convulsion

Point: Duiduan
Meridian: DU 27
Location: On median tubercle of upper lip, at transitional zone between skin of philtrum and upper lip
Posture: Supine
Angle: Oblique puncture
Direction: Upwards
Depth: 5-10 mm
Indications: Manic-depressive psychosis epistaxis, swelling and pain in gum

Point: Yinjiao
Meridian: DU 28
Location: At junction of labal frenum of upper lip and upper gum

Posture: Supine
Angle: Oblique puncture
Direction: Upwards
Depth: 3-5 mm
Indications: Manic-depressive psychosis, masosinusitis, swelling and pain in gum

Point: Heliao
Meridian: LI 19
Location: Directly below lateral border of naris, at level with Shuigou (DU 26)
Posture: Supine
Angle: Perpendicular puncture
Direction: Superficial to deep
Depth: 5-10 mm
Indications: Toothache

Point: Yingxiang
Meridian: LI 20
Location: At midpoint of nasolabial groove, at midpoint of lateral border of ala nasi
Posture: Supine
Angle: Perpendicular puncture
Direction: Upwards medially
Depth: 6-10 mm
Indications: Nasal disorders, paralysis

Point: Juliao
Meridian: ST 3
Location: Directly below pupil, level with lower border of ala nasi, lateral to nasolabial groove
Posture: Supine
Angle: Perpendicular puncture
Direction: Superficial to deep
Depth: 5-10 mm
Indications: Toothache

3. Forehead and Cheek Region

Point: Dicang
Meridian: ST 4
Location: Directly below Sibai, beside angle of mouth

Posture: Supine
Angle: Oblique puncture
Direction: Toward ear
Depth: 10-20 mm
Indications: Facial paralysis, facial spasm

Point: Daying
Meridian: ST 5
Location: In front of angle of mandible, at anterior border of masseteric tuberposity, pulsation point of facial artery
Posture: Supine
Angle: Oblique puncture
Direction: Superficial to deep
Depth: 10-15 mm
Indications: Toothache, gnathospasmus

Point: Jiache
Meridian: ST 6
Location: About one middle finger's breadth anterior and superior to angle of mandible
Posture: Sitting
Angle: Supine
Direction: Perpendicular puncture
Depth: 10-15 mm
Indications: Toothache, trigeminal neuralgia

Point: Xiaguan
Meridian: ST 7
Location: In depression between zygomatic arch and mandibular notch
Posture: Supine
Angle: Perpendicular puncture
Direction: Superficial to deep
Depth: 10-15 mm
Indications: Toothache, facial paralysis, otitis media

Point: Quanliao
Meridian: SI 18
Location: Directly below outer canthus, in depression on lower border of zygoma
Posture: Supine
Angle: Perpendicular puncture
Direction: Superficial to deep
Depth: 5-10 mm
Indications: Toothache, facial paralysis

Point: Chengjiang
Meridian: RN 24
Location: In depression at center of mentolabial groove
Posture: Supine
Angle: Oblique puncture
Direction: Laterally
Depth: 10-15 mm
Indications: Swelling and pain of gum, salivation, manic-depressive psychosis

4. Parietal Region

Point: Naohu
Meridian: DU 17
Location: 2.5 *cun* directly above midpoint of posterior hairline, 1.5 *cun* directly above Fengfu (DU 16)
Posture: Sitting
Angle: Oblique puncture
Direction: Above to below
Depth: 5-10 mm
Indications: Dizziness, rigidity of nape with headache

Point: Qiangjian
Meridian: DU 18
Location: 4 *cun* directly above midpoint of posterior hairline (1.5 *cun* above Naohu)
Posture: Sitting
Angle: Oblique puncture
Direction: Anterior to posterior, left to right
Depth: 5-10 mm
Indications: Manic-depressive psychosis, rigidity of nape

Point: Houding

Meridian: DU 19
Location: 5.5 *cun* directly above midpoint of posterior hairline (3 *cun* above Naohu)
Posture: Sitting
Angle: Oblique puncture
Direction: Superficial to deep
Depth: 5-10 mm
Indications: Headache, dizziness

Point: Baihui
Meridian: DU 20
Location: Midway at line connecting apexes of both ears
Posture: Sitting
Angle: Oblique puncture
Direction: Superficial to deep
Depth: 5-10 mm
Indications: Manic-depressive psychosis, stroke, hysteroptosis, nocturia

Point: Qianding
Meridian: DU 21
Location: 3.5 *cun* directly above midpoint of anterior harline (1.5 *cun* anterior to Baihui)
Posture: Sitting
Angle: Oblique puncture
Direction: Anterior to posterior
Depth: 3-5 mm
Indications: Dizziness, nasosinusitis

Point: Xinhui
Meridian: DU 22
Location: 2 *cun* directly above midpoint of anterior hairline (3 *cun* anterior to Baihui)
Posture: Sitting
Angle: Oblique puncture
Direction: Anterior to posterior
Depth: 5-10 mm
Indications: Dizziness, nasosinusitis, infantile convulsion

Point: Shangxing
Meridian: DU 23
Location: 1 *cun* directly above midpoint of anterior hairline
Posture: Sitting
Angle: Oblique puncture
Direction: Anterior to posterior
Depth: 5-10 mm
Indications: Headache, nasosinusitis, manic-depressive psychosis

Point: Shenting
Meridian: DU 24
Location: 0.5 *cun* directly above midpoint of anterior hairline
Posture: Sitting
Angle: Oblique puncture
Direction: Anterior to posterior
Depth: 5-10 mm
Indications: Headache, insomnia, epilepsy, rhinitis

Point: Meichong
Meridian: BL 3
Location: 0.5 *cun* within hairline, directly above Cuanzhu (BL 2), between Shenting (Du 24) and Qucha (BL 4)
Posture: Sitting
Angle: Horizontal puncture
Direction: Above to below
Depth: 5-10 mm
Indications: Headache, dizziness, epilepsy, nasal obstruction

Point: Qucha
Meridian: BL 4
Location: 1.5 *cun* lateral to point, 0.5 *cun* directly above midpoint of anterior hairline, at junction of median 1/3 and medial 1/3 of line between Shenting (DU 24) and Touwei (ST 8)
Posture: Sitting
Angle: Horizontal puncture
Direction: Anterior to posterior
Depth: 5-10 mm
Indications: Headache, nasal, obstruction, eye disorders

Point: Wuchu
Meridian: BL 5
Location: 1.5 *cun* lateral to point, 1 *cun* directly above midpoint of anterior hairline
Posture: Sitting
Angle: Horizontal puncture
Direction: Anterior to posterior
Depth: 5-10 mm
Indications: Headache, dizziness, epilepsy

Point: Chengguang
Meridian: BL 6
Location: 1.5 *cun* lateral to point, 2.5 *cun* directly above midpoint of anterior hairline
Posture: Sitting
Angle: Horizontal puncture
Direction: Anterior to posterior
Depth: 5-10 mm
Indications: Headache, eye disorders, febrile diseases

Point: Tongtian
Meridian: BL 7
Location: 1.5 *cun* lateral to point, 4 *cun* directly above midpoint of anterior hairline
Posture: Sitting
Angle: Horizontal puncture
Direction: Anterior to posterior
Depth: 5-10 mm
Indications: Headache, nasal obstruction, epistaxis, rhinorrhea with turbid discharge

Point: Luoque
Meridian: BL 8
Location: 1.5 *cun* lateral to point, 5.5 *cun* directly above midpoint of anterior hairline
Posture: Sitting
Angle: Horizontal puncture
Direction: Anterior to posterior
Depth: 5-10 mm
Indications: Headache, nasal obstruction, epistaxis, rhinorrhea with turbid discharge

Point: Yuzhen
Meridian: BL 9
Location: 1.5 *cun* lateral to point, 2.5 *cun* directly above midpoint of posterior hairline, at level with superior border of external occipital protuberance
Posture: Sitting
Angle: Horizontal puncture
Direction: Anterior to posterior
Depth: 5-10 mm
Indications: Headache, nape pain, nasal obstruction, ophthalmalgia

Point: Benshen
Meridian: GB 13
Location: 0.5 *cun* above anterior hairline, 3 *cun* lateral to Shenting (DU 24)
Posture: Sitting
Angle: Horizontal puncture
Direction: Anterior to posterior
Depth: 5-10 mm
Indications: Headache, dizziness, infantile convulsion

Point: Toulingqi
Meridian: GB 15
Location: 0.5 *cun* above anterior hairline, directly above pupil, at midpoint of line connecting Shenting (DU 24) and Touwei (ST 8)
Posture: Sitting
Angle: Horizontal puncture
Direction: Anterior to posterior
Depth: 5-10 mm
Indications: Headache, dizziness, nasal obstruction

Point: Muchuang
Meridian: GB 16
Location: 1.5 *cun* above anterior hairline, 2.25 *cun* lateral to midline of

head

Posture: Sitting

Angle: Horizontal puncture

Direction: Anterior to posterior

Depth: 5-10 mm

Indications: Headache, swelling and pain of the eye, swelling of face

Point: Zhengying

Meridian: GB 17

Location: 2.5 *cun* above anterior hairline, 2.25 *cun* lateral to midline of head

Posture: Sitting

Angle: Horizontal puncture

Direction: Anterior to posterior

Depth: 5-10 mm

Indications: Headache, dizziness, toothache

Point: Chengling

Meridian: GB 18

Location: 4 *cun* above anterior hairline, 2.25 *cun* lateral to midline of head

Posture: Sitting

Angle: Horizontal puncture

Direction: Anterior to posterior

Depth: 5-10 mm

Indications: Headache, dizziness, eye disorders, asal obstruction

Point: Naokong

Meridian: GB 19

Location: On lateral side of superior occipital protuberance, 2.25 *cun* lateral to midline of head

Posture: Sitting

Angle: Horizontal puncture

Direction: Anterior to posterior

Depth: 5-10 mm

Indications: Headache, dizziness, rigidity of nape with headache

Point: Touwei

Meridian: ST 8

Location: 0.5 *cun* above anterior hairline, at corner of forehead, 4.5 *cun*

lateral to midline of head

Posture: Sitting

Angle: Horizontal puncture

Direction: Anterior to posterior

Depth: 15-20 mm

Indications: Headache, dizziness, ophthalmalgia

Point: Shangguan

Meridian: GB 3

Location: In front of ear, directly above Xiaguan (ST 7), and in depression on superior border of zygonatic arch

Posture: Sitting

Angle: Perpendicular puncture

Direction: Superficial to deep

Depth: 15-20 mm

Indications: Tinnitus, deafness, toothache, migraine

Point: Hanyan

Meridian: GB 4

Location: At junction of superior 1/4 and inferior 3/4 of arc line connecting Touwei (ST 8) and Qubin (GB 7)

Posture: Sitting

Angle: Horizontal puncture

Direction: Anterior to posterior

Depth: 10-15 mm

Indications: Migraine, tinnitus, toothache, dizziness

Point: Xuanlu

Meridian: GB 5

Location: At midpoint of arc line connecting Touwei (ST 8) and Qubin (GB 7)

Posture: Sitting

Angle: Horizontal puncture

Direction: Anterior to posterior

Depth: 10-15 mm

Indications: Migraine, eye disorders, toothache

Point: Xuanli

Meridian: GB 6
Location: At junction of superior 3/4 and inferior 1/4 of arc line connecting Touwei (ST 8) and Qubin (GB 7)
Posture: Sitting
Angle: Horizontal puncture
Direction: Anterior to posterior
Depth: 10-15 mm
Indications: Migraine, eye disorders, tinnitus

Point: Qubin
Meridian: GB 7
Location: At junction of line leveling with ear apex and vertical line of posterior border of temple
Posture: Sitting
Angle: Horizontal puncture
Direction: Anterior to posterior
Depth: 10-15 mm
Indications: Headache, toothache, gnathospasmus

Point: Shuaigu
Meridian: GB 8
Location: Directly above ear apex, and 1.5 *cun* within hairline, directly above Jiaosun (SJ 20)
Posture: Sitting
Angle: Horizontal puncture
Direction: Anterior to posterior
Depth: 10-15 mm
Indications: Migraine, dizziness, infantile convulsion

Point: Tianchong
Meridian: GB 9
Location: 2 *cun* within hairline and directly above posterior border of auricular, 0.5 *cun* posterior to Shuaigu (GB 8)
Posture: Sitting
Angle: Horizontal puncture
Direction: Anterior to posterior
Depth: 10-15 mm

Indications: Headache, manic-depressive psychosis, swelling and pain of gum

Point: Heliao
Meridian: SJ 22
Location: At lateral aspect of head and posterior border of temple, in front of auricle and posterior border of superficial temporal artery
Posture: Sitting
Angle: Oblique or horizontal puncture
Direction: Anterior to posterior
Depth: 15-20 mm
Indications: Headache, tinnitus, gnathospasmus

5. Auricular Region

Point: Tinggong
Meridian: SI 19
Location: On face, in front of tragus, in depression and posterior border of amndibular condy loid process when opening mouth
Posture: Sitting
Angle: Perpendicular puncture
Direction: Superficial to deep
Depth: 15-20 mm
Indications: Deafness, otalgia

Point: Tinghui
Meridian: GB 2
Location: In front of intertragicnotch, in depression and posterior border of mandibular condy loid process when opening mouth
Posture: Sitting
Angle: Perpendicular puncture
Direction: Superficial to deep
Depth: 10-15 mm
Indications: Otopathy, toothache, facial paralysis

Point: Yifeng
Meridian: SJ 17
Location: At posterior to ear lobe, and

in depression between angle of mandible and mastoid process

Posture: Sitting
Angle: Perpendicular puncture
Direction: Superficial to deep
Depth: 15-20 mm
Indications: Otitis media, tinnitus

Point: Chimai
Meridian: SJ 18
Location: At center of mastoid process, between Jiaosun (SJ 20) and Yifeng (SJ 17), and at junction of median 1/3 and inferior 1/3 of line along helix
Posture: Sitting
Angle: Horizontal puncture
Direction: Anterior to posterior
Depth: 5-10 mm
Indications: Headache, tinnitus

Point: Luxi
Meridian: SJ 19
Location: At posterior to ear, between Jiaosun (SJ 20) and Yifeng (SJ 17), at junction of superior 1/3 and median 1/3 of line alone helix
Posture: Sitting
Angle: Horizontal puncture
Direction: Anterior to posterior
Depth: 5-10 mm
Indications: Headache, tinnitus

Point: Jiaosun
Meridian: SJ 20
Location: In hairline directly above apex auricular
Posture: Sitting
Angle: Horizontal puncture
Direction: Above to below
Depth: 5-10 mm
Indications: Toothache, migraine

Point: Fubai
Meridian: GB 10
Location: At superior and posterior to mastoid process, at junction of median 1/3 and superior 1/3 of arc line between Tianchong (GB 9) and Wangu (GB 12)
Posture: Sitting
Angle: Oblique puncture
Direction: Above to below
Depth: 5-10 mm
Indications: Headache, deafness

Point: Touqiaoyin
Meridian: GB 11
Location: At superior and posterior to mastoid process, at junction of median 1/3 and inferior 1/3 of arc line between Tianchong (GB 9) and Wangu (GB 12)
Posture: Sitting
Angle: Horizontal puncture
Direction: Above to below
Depth: 10-15 mm
Indications: Headache, deafness, tinnitus

Point: Wangu
Meridian: GB 12
Location: In depression posterior and inferior to mastoid process
Posture: Sitting
Angle: Oblique puncture
Direction: Toward contralateral orbit
Depth: 20-30 mm
Indications: Headache, rigidity of nape with headache, malaria, toothache

Point: Ermen
Meridian: SJ
Location: In front of supratragic notch of auricle and at depression when opening mouth
Posture: Sitting
Angle: Perpendicular puncture
Direction: Superficial to deep
Depth: 10-20 mm
Indications: Deafness, toothache, tinnitus

6. Nape Region

Point: Fengchi
Meridian: GB 20
Location: Below occipital bone, on level with Fengfu (DU 16) and at depression between sternocleidomastoid muscle and trapezius muscle
Posture: Sitting
Angle: Oblique puncture
Direction: Toward nasal apex
Depth: 10-20 mm
Indications: Headache, omalgia, cold, eye disorders

Point: Tianzhu
Meridian: BL 10
Location: On nape, at depression within posterior hairline and lateral border of trapezius muscle, 1.3 *cun* lateral to posterior midline
Posture: Sitting
Angle: Perpendicular puncture
Direction: Toward orbit
Depth: 10-20 mm
Indications: Headache, nasal obstruction, nape pain, omalgia

Point: Yamen
Meridian: DU 15
Location: 0.5 *cun* directly above midpoint of posterior hairline and below first cervical vertebra
Posture: Sitting
Angle: Perpendicular puncture
Direction: Down toward oral part
Depth: 10-20 mm
Indications: Deaf-mutism, schizophrenia, headache

Point: Fengfu
Meridian: DU 16
Location: 1 *cun* directly above midpoint of posterior hairline and at depression between both trapezius muscles
Posture: Sitting
Angle: Perpendicular puncture
Direction: Posterior to anterior
Depth: 10-20 mm
Indications: Headache, nape pain, manic-depressive psychosis, apoplexy

7. Anterior Cervical Region

Point: Tiantu
Meridian: RN 22
Location: At center of suprasternal fossa
Posture: Sitting
Angle: Perpendicular puncture
Direction: Toward posterior of sternum
Depth: 20-30 mm
Indications: Asthma, cough

Point: Lianquan
Meridian: RN 23
Location: On anterior midline and above Adam's apple, at depression on superior border of hyoid bone
Posture: Sitting
Angle: Oblique puncture
Direction: Toward root of tongue
Depth: 10-20 mm
Indications: Aphasia, dysphagia

Point: Renying
Meridian: ST 9
Location: Lateral to Adam's apple and at anterior border of sternocleidomastoid muscle, about where common carotid artery is palpable
Posture: Sitting
Angle: Perpendicular puncture
Direction: Superficial to deep, avoiding artery
Depth: 10-20 mm
Indications: Asthma, hypertension

Point: Shuitu

Meridian: ST 10
Location: Between Renying (ST 9) and Qishe (ST 11), at anterior border of sternocleidomastoid muscle
Posture: Sitting
Angle: Perpendicular puncture
Direction: Superficial to deep
Depth: 10-20 mm
Indications: Swelling and sore throat, asthma

Point: Qishe
Meridian: ST 11
Location: At superior border of medial end of clavicle, and between sternal head and clavicular head of the sternocleidomastoid muscle
Posture: Sitting
Angle: Perpendicular puncture
Direction: Superficial to deep
Depth: 5-10 mm
Indications: Asthma, nape pain, vegetative nerve functional disturbance

Point: Quepen
Meridian: ST 12
Location: At center of supraclavicular fossa, 4 *cun* lateral to anterior midline of the chest
Posture: Sitting
Angle: Perpendicular puncture
Direction: Superficial to deep
Depth: 5-10 mm
Indications: Cough, asthma, swelling and sore throat

Point: Tianding
Meridian: LI 17
Location: Lateral to Adam's apple and at posterior border of sternocleidomastoid muscle, between Futu (LI 18) and Quepen (ST 12)
Posture: Sitting
Angle: Perpendicular puncture
Direction: Superficial to deep
Depth: 10-15 mm

Indications: Swelling and sore throat, tonsillitis

Point: Futu
Meridian: LI 18
Location: Lateral to Adam's apple, and between posterior border and anterior border of sternocleidomastoid muscle
Posture: Sitting
Angle: Perpendicular puncture
Direction: Superficial to deep
Depth: 10-15 mm
Indications: Hoarseness, goiter

Point: Tianchuang
Meridian: SI 16
Location: At posterior border of sternoclei-domastoid muscle and level with Adam's apple, posterior to Futu (LI 18)
Posture: Sitting
Angle: Perpendicular puncture
Direction: Superficial to deep
Depth: 10-20 mm
Indications: Tinnitus, swelling and sore throat

Point: Tianrong
Meridian: SI 17
Location: Posterior to angle of mandible, and in depression on anterior border of sternocleidomastoid muscle
Posture: Sitting
Angle: Perpendicular puncture
Direction: Superficial to deep
Depth: 15-25 mm
Indications: Tonsillitis, swelling and pain of neck and nape

Point: Tianyou
Meridian: SJ 16
Location: Directly below posterior to mastoid process and level with angle of mandible, at posterior border of sternocleidomastoid muscle

Posture: Sitting
Angle: Perpendicular puncture
Direction: Superficial to deep
Depth: 15-25 mm
Indications: Headache, swelling of face, migraine

8. Anterior Aspect of Upper Arm

Point: Tianfu
Meridian: LU 3
Location: On medial aspect of arm and radial border of biceps brachii, 3 *cun* below end of anterior axillary fold
Posture: Sitting
Angle: Perpendicular puncture
Direction: External to interior
Depth: 10-15 mm
Indications: Asthma, epistaxis

Point: Xiabai
Meridian: LU 4
Location: On medial aspect of arm and radial border of biceps brachii, 4 *cun* below end of anterior axillary fold
Posture: Sitting
Angle: Perpendicular puncture
Direction: External to interior
Depth: 10-15 mm
Indications: Cough, pectoralgia

Point: Tianquan
Meridian: PC 2
Location: On medial aspect of arm, 2 *cun* below head of anterior axillary fold, between two-heads of biceps brachii
Posture: Sitting
Angle: Perpendicular puncture
Direction: External to deep
Depth: 15-20 mm
Indications: Pain in chest, and hypochondrium, cough

Point: Jiquan
Meridian: HT 1
Location: At center of axillary fossa, where axillary artery is palpable
Posture: Lateral recumbent
Angle: Perpendicular puncture
Direction: Superficial to deep
Depth: 10-15 mm
Indications: Pain in hypochondriac region, cardalgia

Point: Qingling
Meridian: HT 2
Location: On medial aspect of arm and line connecting Jiquan (HT 1) and Shaohai (HT 3), 3 *cun* above cubital crease, the medial side of bicpes brachii
Posture: Sitting
Angle: Perpendicular puncture
Direction: Superficial to deep
Depth: 10-20 mm
Indications: Jaundice, hypochondriac pain

9. Angerior Aspect of Forearm

Point: Chize
Meridian: LU 5
Location: On cubital crease, in depression on radial side of tendon of biceps brachii
Posture: Sitting
Angle: Perpendicular puncture
Direction: Superficial to deep
Depth: 10-15 mm
Indications: Cough, hymoptysis, tidal fever, asthma

Point: Kongzui
Meridian: LU 6
Location: On line joining Taiyuan (LU 9) and Chize (Lu 5), and 7 *cun* above transverse crease of wrist
Posture: Sitting
Angle: Perpendicular puncture

Direction: Superficial to deep
Depth: 10-20 mm
Indications: Cough, asthma, hemoptysis, hemorrhoids

Point: Lieque
Meridian: LU 7
Location: Superior to styloid process of radius, 1.5 *cun* above transverse crease of wrist, and between brachioradial muscle and tendon of long abductor muscle of thumb
Posture: Sitting
Angle: Oblique puncture
Direction: Toward cubitus
Depth: 5-10 mm
Indications: Headache, cough, asthma, pain of inferior tooth

Point: Jingqu
Meridian: LU 8
Location: In depression between radial artery and styloid process of radius
Posture: Sitting
Angle: Perpendicular puncture
Direction: Superficial to deep
Depth: 5-10 mm
Indications: Cough, asthma, pectoralgia

Point: Taiyuan
Meridian: LU 9
Location: At radial end of crease of wrist, where radial artery is palpable
Posture: Sitting
Angle: Perpendicular puncture
Direction: Superficial to deep
Depth: 5-10 mm
Indications: Cough, asthma, pectoralgia

Point: Quze
Meridian: PC 3
Location: On transverse cubital crease, at ulnar side of tendon of the biceps brachii
Posture: Sitting

Angle: Perpendicular puncture
Direction: Superficial to deep
Depth: 10-20 mm
Indications: Cardialgia, stomachalgia, febrile disease, diarrhea

Point: Ximen
Meridian: PC 4
Location: Between Quze (PC 3) and Daling (PC 7), 5 *cun* above transverse crease of wrist
Posture: Sitting
Angle: Perpendicular puncture
Direction: Superficial to deep
Depth: 15-20 mm
Indications: Cardialgia, hematemesis, furuncle, palpitation

Point: Jianshi
Meridian: PC 5
Location: On line connecting Quze (PC 3) and Daling (PC 7), 3 *cun* above transverse crease of wrist
Posture: Sitting
Angle: Perpendicular puncture
Direction: Superficial to deep
Depth: 15-20 mm
Indications: Cardialgia, stomachalgia, febrile disease, malaria

Point: Neiguan
Meridian: PC 6
Location: On line connecting Quze (PC 3) and Daling (PC 7), 2 *cun* above transverse crease of wrist
Posture: Sitting
Angle: Perpendicular puncture
Direction: Superficial to deep
Depth: 15-20 mm
Indications: Arrhythmia, shock, hypertension, hysteria, angiitis

Point: Daling
Meridian: PC 7
Location: At middle of transverse crease of wrist, between crease of wrist, between tendons of long pal-

mar muscle and radial flexor muscle of wrist

Posture: Sitting
Angle: Perpendicular puncture
Direction: Superficial to deep
Depth: 10-15 mm
Indications: Palpitation, stomachalgia, insomnia, manic-depressive psychosis

Point: Shaohai
Meridian: HT 3
Location: When the elbow is flexed, point is between medial end of transverse cubital crease and media epicondyle of humerus
Posture: Sitting
Angle: Perpendicular puncture
Direction: Superficial to deep
Depth: 15-20 mm
Indications: Cardialgia, head tremor, hypochondriac pain

Point: Lingdao
Meridian: HT 4
Location: On lateral border of tendon of ulnar flexor muscle of wrist, and 1.5 *cun* above transverse crease of wrist
Posture: Sitting
Angle: Perpendicular puncture
Direction: Superficial to deep
Depth: 6-10 mm
Indications: Cardiopathy, hysteria

Point: Tongli
Meridian: HT 5
Location: On lateral border of tendon of ulnar flexor muscle of wrist, and 1 *cun* above transverse crease of wrist
Posture: Sitting
Angle: Perpendicular puncture
Direction: Superficial to deep
Depth: 6-10 mm
Indications: Palpitation, insomnia,

aphasis
Point: Yinxi
Meridian: HT 6
Location: On lateral border of tendon of ulnar flexor muscle of wrist, and 0.5 *cun* above transverse crease of wrist
Posture: Sitting
Angle: Perpendicular puncture
Direction: Superficial to deep
Depth: 5-10 mm
Indications: Palpitation, night sweats

Point: Shenmen
Meridian: HT 7
Location: On wrist and radial side of tendon of ulnar flexor muscle of wrist, at medial end of transverse crease of wrist
Posture: Sitting
Angle: Perpendicular puncture
Direction: Superficial to deep
Depth: 5-10 mm
Indications: Insomnia, manic-depressive psychosis, palpitation, hysteria

10. Anterior Aspect of Hand

Point: Yuji
Meridian: LU 10
Location: On radial aspect of midpoint of first metacarpal bone, on junction of red and white skin nail
Posture: Sitting
Angle: Perpendicular puncture
Direction: Superficial to deep
Depth: 10-15 mm
Indications: Cough, swollen and sore throat, fever

Point: Shaoshang
Meridian: LU 11
Location: On radial side of tip of thumb, 0.1 *cun* proximal to nail
Posture: Sitting
Angle: Horizontal puncture

Direction: Superficial to deep
Depth: 3 mm
Indications: Laryngalgia, fever, respiratory failure, apoplexy

Point: Laogong
Meridian: PC 8
Location: At part touching tip of middle finger when making fist
Posture: Sitting
Angle: Perpendicular puncture
Direction: Superficial to deep
Depth: 5-10 mm
Indications: Cardialgia, vomiting, aphtha, ozostomia

Point: Zhongchong
Meridian: PC 3
Location: At center of tip of middle finger
Posture: Sitting
Angle: Perpendicular puncture
Direction: Toward anterior aspect of digitus
Depth: 3 mm
Indications: Heliosis, spoplexy, infantile convulsion, coma

Point: Shaofu
Meridian: HT 8
Location: At point touching tip of little finger when making fist
Posture: Sitting
Angle: Perpendicular puncture
Direction: From superficial to deep
Depth: 5-10 mm
Indications: Palpitation, enuresis, pectoralgia

Point: Shaochong
Meridian: HT 9
Location: On radial side of tip of little finger, 0.1 *cun* proximal to corner of nail
Posture: Sitting
Angle: Horizontal puncture
Direction: Superficial to deep

Depth: 3 mm
Indications: Palpitation, febrile disease, coma

11. Posterior Aspect of Upper Arm

Point: Zhouliao
Meridian: LI 12
Location: When elbow flexed, 1 *cun* above Quchi (LI 11), and on lateral border of lateral epicondyle of humerus
Posture: Sitting
Angle: Oblique puncture
Direction: Toward forearm
Depth: 10-20 mm
Indications: Pain in elbow and arm, numbness of upper limb

Point: Shouwuli
Meridian: LI 13
Location: On lateral aspect of arm and 3 *cun* above Quchi (LI 11), at line connecting Quchi and Jianyu (LI 15)
Posture: Sitting
Angle: Perpendicular puncture
Direction: Medial to lateral aspect
Depth: 15-20 mm
Indications: Pain in elbow and arm, tuberculosis of lymph nodes

Point: Binao
Meridian: LI 14
Location: On lateral aspect of arm and 7 *cun* above Quchi (LI 11), in line connecting Quchi and Jianyu (LI 15) at insertion of deltoid muscle
Posture: Sitting
Angle: Perpendicular puncture
Direction: Toward joint
Depth: 15-20 mm
Indications: Disorders of the shoulder and arm, urticaria

Point: Jianyu
Meridian: LI 15
Location: On deltoid muscle, when arm fully abducted, in depression inferior and anterior to acromion
Posture: Sitting
Angle: Perpendicular puncture
Direction: Toward joint
Depth: 30-40 mm
Indications: Paraplegia superior, disorders of joint and soft tissue

Point: Tianjing
Meridian: SJ 10
Location: On lateral aspect of arm, when elbow flexed, about 1 *cun* directly above olecranon
Posture: Sitting
Angle: Perpendicular puncture
Direction: Lateral to medial aspect
Depth: 10-20 mm
Indications: Disorders of elbow, tuberculosis of lymph nodes

Point: Qinglengyuan
Meridian: SJ 11
Location: On lateral aspect of arm and 1 *cun* above Tianjing (SJ 10), 2 *cun* directly above olecranon
Posture: Sitting
Angle: Perpendicular puncture
Direction: Lateral to medial aspect
Depth: 8-10 mm
Indications: Pain in shoulder and arm

Point: Xiaoluo
Meridian: SJ 12
Location: On lateral aspect of arm, at midpoint of line connecting Qinglengyuan (SJ 11) and Naohui (SJ 13)
Posture: Sitting
Angle: Perpendicular puncture
Direction: Lateral to medial aspect
Depth: 10-15 mm
Indications: Headache rigidity of nape and neck, brachial palsy

Point: Naohui
Meridian: SJ 13
Location: In posteroinferior border of deltoid muscle, 3 *cun* below Jianliao (SJ 14), on line joining Jianliao (SJ 14) and tip of olecranon
Posture: Sitting
Angle: Perpendicular puncture
Direction: Lateral to medial aspect
Depth: 15-10 mm
Indications: Omalgia, eye disorders

Point: Jianliao
Meridian: SJ 14
Location: Posterior to Jianyu (LI 15) when arm in full abduction, in depression on posteroinferior to acromion
Posture: Sitting
Angle: Perpendicular puncture
Direction: Toward shoulder joint
Depth: 15-20 mm
Indications: Brachialgia, paraplegia superior

Point: Jianzhen
Meridian: SJ 9
Location: Posteroinferior to shoulder joint, when arm abducted, 1 *cun* above posterior end of axillary fold
Posture: Sitting
Angle: Perpendicular puncture
Direction: Toward shoulder joint
Depth: 15-20 mm
Indications: Omalgia, pain in hand and arm

12. Posterior Aspect of Hand

Point: Yangxi
Meridian: LI 5
Location: On radial side of carpel transverse crease when thumb tilted upward, between tendons of long extensor and short extensor muscles

of thumb
Posture: Sitting
Angle: Perpendicular puncture
Direction: Lateral to medial aspect
Depth: 8-10 mm
Indications: Headache, deafness, toothache, sore throat

Point: Pianli
Meridian: LI 6
Location: On radial side of posterior aspect of forearm, in line joining Yangxi (LI 5) and Quchi (LI 11), 3 *cun* above transverse crease of wrist
Posture: Sitting
Angle: Perpendicular puncture
Direction: Lateral to medial aspect
Depth: 10-15 mm
Indications: Epistaxis, deafness, hydrops

Point: Wenliu
Meridian: LI 7
Location: On radial side of posterior aspect of forearm, in line joining Yangxi (LI 5) and Quchi (LI 11), 5 *cun* above transverse crease of wrist
Posture: Sitting
Angle: Perpendicular puncture
Direction: Lateral to medial aspect
Depth: 10-15 mm
Indications: Headache, sore throat

Point: Xialiao
Meridian: LI 8
Location: On radial side of posterior aspect of forearm, in line joining Yangxi (LI 5) and Quchi (LI 11), 4 *cun* below transverse cubital crease
Posture: Sitting
Angle: Perpendicular puncture
Direction: Lateral to medial aspect
Depth: 10-15 mm
Indications: Pain in elbow and arm, abdominalgia

Point: Shanglian

Meridian: LI 9
Location: On radial side of posterior aspect of forearm, in line joining Yangxi (LI 5) and Quchi (LI 11), 3 *cun* below transverse cubital crease
Posture: Sitting
Angle: Perpendicular puncture
Direction: Lateral to medial aspect
Depth: 10-15 mm
Indications: Pain in shoulder and arm, vomiting, diarrhea, paraplegia superior

Point: Shousanli
Meridian: LI 10
Location: On radial side of posterior aspect of forearm, in line joining Yangxi (LI 5) and Quchi (LI 11), 2 *cun* below transverse cubital crease
Posture: Sitting
Angle: Perpendicular puncture
Direction: Lateral to medial aspect
Depth: 10-15 mm
Indications: Pain in shoulder and arm, vomiting, diarrhea, paraplegia

Point: Quchi
Meridian: LI 11
Location: At lateral end of transverse cubital crease when elbow flexed, at midpoint of line joining Chize (LU 57) and lateral epicondyle of humerus
Posture: Sitting
Angle: Perpendicular puncture
Direction: Lateral to medial aspect
Depth: 10-20 mm
Indications: Hypertension, fever, paraplegia superior, urticaria

Point: Yangchi
Meridian: SJ 4
Location: At lateral end of transverse crease of wrist, in depression on ulnar border of extensor tendon of finger

Posture: Sitting
Angle: Perpendicular puncture
Direction: Toward joint
Depth: 5-10 mm
Indications: Chronic diseases of digestive system, deafness, eye disorders

Point: Waiguan
Meridian: SJ 5
Location: On line joining Yangchi (SJ 4) and tip of oleranon, 2 *cun* above transverse crease of wrist and between radius and ulna
Posture: Sitting
Angle: Perpendicular puncture
Direction: Dorsum to palm
Depth: 15-20 mm
Indications: Paraplegia superior, stiff neck, deafness, febrile disease

Point: Zhigou
Meridian: SJ 6
Location: On line joining Yangchi (SJ 4) and tip of olecranon, 3 *cun* above transverse crease of wrist and between radius and ulna
Posture: Sitting
Angle: Perpendicular puncture
Direction: Dorsum to palm
Depth: 15-20 mm
Indications: Constipation, sore throat, deafness, pain in shoulder and back

Point: Huizong
Meridian: SJ 7
Location: 3 *cun* above transverse crease of wrist and between radius and ulna on ulna side to Zhigou (SJ 6)
Posture: Sitting
Angle: Perpendicular puncture
Direction: Dorsum to palm
Depth: 10-15 mm
Indications: Deafness, pain of upper limb, epilepsy

Point: Sanyangluo
Meridian: SJ 8

Location: 4 *cun* above transverse crease of wrist and between radius and ulna on ulna side to Zhigou (SJ 6)
Posture: Sitting
Angle: Perpendicular puncture
Direction: Dorsum to palm
Depth: 10-15 mm
Indications: Deafness, aphasia

Point: Sidu
Meridian: SJ 9
Location: On posterior aspect of forearm in line joining Yangchi (SJ 4) and tip of olecranon, 5 *cun* below the tip of olecranon between radius and ulna
Posture: Sitting
Angle: Perpendicular puncture
Direction: Dorsum to palm
Depth: 15-20 mm
Indications: Deafness, pain of forearm, toothache

Point: Yanggu
Meridian: SI 5
Location: On ulnar side of the wrist, in depression between styloid process of ulna and triquetral bone
Posture: Sitting
Angle: Perpendicular puncture
Direction: Toward joint
Depth: 5-10 mm
Indications: Febrile disease, pain of ulna nerve

Point: Yanglao
Meridian: SI 6
Location: On posterior aspect of forearm, in depression on radial side of proximal end of ulna
Posture: Sitting
Angle: Oblique puncture
Direction: Upward
Depth: 5-10 mm
Indications: Ophthalmocopia, brachial neuralgia

Point: Zhizheng
Meridian: SI 7
Location: On ulnar side of posterior aspect of forearm, on line joining Yanggu (SI 5) and Xiaohai (SI 8), 5 *cun* above transverse crease of wrist
Posture: Sitting
Angle: Perpendicular puncture
Direction: Dorsum to palm
Depth: 5-10 mm
Indications: Rigidity of nape, febrile disease, neuralgia

Point: Xiaohai
Meridian: SI 8
Location: On medial side of elbow and in depression between olecranon of ulna and medial epicondyle of humerus
Posture: Sitting
Angle: Perpendicular puncture
Direction: Into joint
Depth: 5-10 mm
Indications: Pain of nape, neck and shoulder, epilepsy, tinnitus

13. Dorsum of Hand

Point: Shangyang
Meridian: LI 1
Location: On radial side of index finger, 0.1 *cun* proximal to corner of nail
Posture: Sitting
Angle: Perpendicular puncture
Direction: Toward anterior aspect of finger
Depth: 3 mm
Indications: Deafness, toothache, febrile disease, apoplexy

Point: Erjian
Meridian: LI 2
Location: When fist made slightly, distal to second metacarpophalangeal joint, in depression on radial side

Posture: Sitting
Angle: Perpendicular puncture
Direction: From radius to ulna
Depth: 5-8 mm
Indications: Epistaxis, facial paralysis, febrile disease

Point: Sanjian
Meridian: LI 3
Location: When fist made slightly, proximal to second metacarpophalangeal joint, in depression on radial side
Posture: Sitting
Angle: Perpendicular puncture
Direction: Radius to ulna
Depth: 5-8 mm
Indications: Ophthalmalgia, toothache, sore throat

Point: Hegu
Meridian: LI 4
Location: Between first and second metacarpal bones, at midpoint of radial side of second metacarpal bone
Posture: Sitting
Angle: Perpendicular puncture
Direction: Dorsum to palm
Depth: 8-10 mm
Indications: Headache, toothache, amenorrhea, prolonged labor

Point: Guanchong
Meridian: SJ 1
Location: On ulnar side of ring finger, 0.1 *cun* proximal to corner of nail
Posture: Sitting
Angle: Perpendicular puncture
Direction: Toward anterior aspect of finger
Depth: 3-5 mm
Indications: Headache, stiff tongue, febrile disease, vexation

Point: Yemen
Meridian: SJ 2
Location: Between ring and little fin-

ger, proximal to finger web between red and white skin
Posture: Sitting
Angle: Perpendicular puncture
Direction: Dorsum to palm
Depth: 5-10 mm
Indications: Headache, coma, malaria, shock

Point: Zhongzhu
Meridian: SJ 3
Location: Between fourth and fifth metacarpal bones, in depression proximal to fourth metacarpophalangeal joint
Posture: Sitting
Angle: Perpendicular puncture
Direction: Dorsum to palm
Depth: 5-10 mm
Indications: Headache, deafness, vomiting, blurred vision

Point: Shaoze
Meridian: SI 11
Location: On ulnar side of little finger, 0.1 *cun* proximal to corner of nail
Posture: Sitting
Angle: Oblique puncture
Direction: Toward anterior aspect of finger
Depth: 3-5 mm
Indications: Febrile disease, coma, hypogalactia

Point: Qiangu
Meridian: SI 2
Location: On ulnar border of hand and transverse crease end distal to fifth metacarpophalangeal joint
Posture: Sitting
Angle: Oblique puncture
Direction: Ulna to radius
Depth: 5-10 mm
Indications: Brachialgia, numbness of little finger, febrile disease

Point: Houxi

Meridian: SI 3
Location: On ulnar border of palm, when loose fist made, at transverse crease end of palm proximal to fifth metacarpophalangeal joint, at junction of red and white skin
Posture: Sitting
Angle: Oblique puncture
Direction: Ulna to radius
Depth: 5-10 mm
Indications: Disorders of head and nape, eye disorders, epilepsy

Point: Wangu
Meridian: SI 4
Location: On the ulnar border of palm and between base of fifth metacarpal and hamate bones
Posture: Sitting
Angle: Perpendicular puncture
Direction: Ulna to radius
Depth: 5-10 mm
Indications: Stiff nape, eye disorders, jaundice, febrile diseases

14. Chest

Point: Zhongting
Meridian: RN 16
Location: On anterior midline of thorax at junction of body of sternum and xiphoid process, level with fifth intercostal space
Posture: Supine
Angle: Oblique puncture
Direction: Upward
Depth: 5-10 mm
Indications: Cholecystitis, vomiting of milk, dysphagia

Point: Dazhong
Meridian: RN 17
Location: On anterior midline of thorax, level with fourth intercostal space, midway between nipples
Posture: Supine

Angle: Oblique puncture
Direction: Downward
Depth: 8-10 mm
Indications: Asthma, bronchitis, pectoralgia, hypogalactia

Point: Yutang
Meridian: RN 18
Location: On anterior midline of thorax, level with third intercostal space
Posture: Supine
Angle: Oblique puncture
Direction: Downward
Depth: 10-15 mm
Indications: Cough, asthma, pectoralgia

Point: Zigong
Meridian: RN 19
Location: On anterior midline of thorax, level with second intercostal space
Posture: Supine
Angle: Oblique puncture
Direction: Downward
Depth: 8-10 mm
Indications: Cough, asthma, pectoralgia

Point: Huagai
Meridian: RN 20
Location: On anterior midline of thorax, level with first intercostal space
Posture: Supine
Angle: Oblique puncture
Direction: Downward
Depth: 8-10 mm
Indications: Cough, asthma, pectoralgia

Point: Xuanji
Meridian: RN 21
Location: On anterior midline of thorax, 1 *cun* below Tiantu (RN 22)
Posture: Supine
Angle: Oblique puncture
Direction: Downward

Depth: 8-10 mm
Indications: Cough, asthma, pectoralgia

Point: Bulang
Meridian: KI 22
Location: In fifth intercostal space, 2 *cun* lateral to the anterior midline
Posture: Sitting
Angle: Perpendicular puncture
Direction: Toward intercostal space
Depth: 10-15 mm
Indications: Cough, asthma

Point: Shenfeng
Meridian: KI 23
Location: In fourth intercostal space, 2 *cun* lateral to anterior midline
Posture: Sitting
Angle: Perpendicular puncture
Direction: Toward intercostal space
Depth: 10-15 mm
Indications: Mastitis, full sensation in chest, asthma

Point: Lingxu
Meridian: KI 24
Location: In third intercostal space, 2 *cun* lateral to anterior midline
Posture: Supine
Angle: Perpendicular puncture
Direction: Toward intercostal space
Depth: 10-15 mm
Indications: Mastitis, pleuritis

Point: Shencang
Meridian: KI 25
Location: In second intercostal space, 2 *cun* lateral to anterior midline
Posture: Supine
Angle: Perpendicular puncture
Direction: Toward intercostal space
Depth: 5-10 mm
Indications: Arteriosclerosis, pectoralgia

Point: Yuzhong
Meridian: KI 26

Location: In first intercostal space, 2 *cun* lateral to anterior midline
Posture: Supine
Angle: Perpendicular puncture
Direction: Toward intercostal space
Depth: 5-10 mm
Indications: Heart disorders, bronchitis

Point: Shufu
Meridian: KI 27
Location: On inferior border of clavicle, 2 *cun* lateral to anterior midline
Posture: Supine
Angle: Perpendicular puncture
Direction: Toward intercostal space
Depth: 5-10 mm
Indications: Heart diseases, cough, asthma

Point: Qihu
Meridian: ST 13
Location: At inferior border of midpoint of clavicle, 4 *cun* lateral to anterior midline
Posture: Sitting
Angle: Oblique puncture
Direction: Toward shoulder
Depth: 10-15 mm
Indications: Cold, trachitis, mastitis

Point: Kufang
Meridian: ST 14
Location: In first intercostal space, 4 *cun* lateral to anterior midline
Posture: Sitting
Angle: Oblique puncture
Direction: Toward shoulder
Depth: 10-15 mm
Indications: Distending pain in hypochondrium, cough

Point: Wuyi
Meridian: ST 15
Location: In second intercostal space, 4 *cun* lateral to anterior midline
Posture: Sitting
Angle: Oblique puncture

Direction: Toward shoulder
Depth: 10-15 mm
Indications: Mastitis, cough, pectoralgia

Point: Yingchuang
Meridian: ST 16
Location: In third intercostal space, 4 *cun* lateral to anterior midline
Posture: Sitting
Angle: Oblique puncture
Direction: Toward shoulder
Depth: 10-15 mm
Indications: Mastitis, cough, pectoralgia

Point: Ruzhong
Meridian: ST 17
Location: In fourth intercostal space, 4 *cun* lateral to anterior midline, at center of nipple
Posture: Sitting
Angle: Oblique puncture
Direction: Toward shoulder
Depth: 10-15 mm
Indications: Do not puncture with needle

Point: Rugen
Meridian: ST 18
Location: In fourth intercostal space, 4 *cun* lateral to anterior midline, directly below nipple, on lower border of breast
Posture: Sitting
Angle: Oblique puncture
Direction: Toward shoulder
Depth: 10-15 mm
Indications: Hypogalactia, mastitis, heart diseases

Point: Zhongfu
Meridian: LU 1
Location: 1 *cun* below Yunmen (LU 2), level with first intercostal space, 6 *cun* lateral to anterior midline
Posture: Supine

Angle: Perpendicular puncture
Direction: Chest to back, slightly laterally
Depth: 15-20 mm
Indications: Cough, asthma, tuberculosis of lung

Point: Yunmen
Meridian: LU 2
Location: On superior and lateral aspect of anterior pectoral region, superior to coracoid process of scapula, in depression on infraclavicular fossa, 6 *cun* lateral to anterior midline
Posture: Sitting
Angle: Perpendicular puncture
Direction: Chest to back, slightly laterally
Depth: 15-20 mm
Indications: Cough, asthma, tuberculosis of lung

Point: Shourong
Meridian: SP 20
Location: Lateral region of chest, in second intercostal space, 6 *cun* lateral to anterior midline
Posture: Sitting
Angle: Oblique puncture
Direction: Toward intercostal space
Depth: 8-10 mm
Indications: Pain in chest and ribs, cough

Point: Dabao
Meridian: SP 21
Location: Lateral region of chest and on mid-axillary line, in sixth intercostal space
Posture: Prone
Angle: Oblique puncture
Direction: Toward intercostal space
Depth: 10-15 mm
Indications: Cough, asthma, oppressed feeling in chest, brachial palsy

Point: Yuanye
Meridian: GB 22
Location: Lateral region of chest. When arm raised, on mid-axillary line and 3 *cun* below axilla in fourth intercostal space
Posture: Sitting
Angle: Oblique puncture
Direction: Toward intercostal space
Depth: 10-15 mm
Indications: Intercostal neuralgia

Point: Zhejin
Meridian: GB 23
Location: Lateral region of chest, 1 *cun* anterior to Yuanye (GB 22), level with nipple, in fourth intercostal space
Posture: Lateral recumbent
Angle: Oblique puncture
Direction: Toward intercostal space
Depth: 8-10 mm
Indications: Full sensation in chest, asthma

Point: Shidou
Meridian: SP 17
Location: 6 *cun* lateral to anterior midline in fifth intercostal space
Posture: Supine
Angle: Oblique puncture
Direction: Toward intercostal space
Depth: 8-10 mm
Indications: Dysphagia, distending pain in the chest and ribs

Point: Tianxi
Meridian: SP 18
Location: Lateral side of chest, in fourth intercostal space, 6 *cun* lateral to anterior midline
Posture: Supine
Angle: Oblique puncture
Direction: Toward intercostal space
Depth: 8-10 mm
Indications: Pectoralgia, cough, hypo-

galactia

Point: Xiongxiang
Meridian: SP 19
Location: Lateral side of chest, in third intercostal space, 6 *cun* lateral to anterior midline
Posture: Supine
Angle: Oblique puncture
Direction: Toward intercostal space
Depth: 8-10 mm
Indications: Pleuritis, distending pain in the chest and rib

Point: Tianchi
Meridian: PC 1
Location: 1 *cun* lateral to nipple, in fourth intercostal space, 5 *cun* lateral to anterior midline
Posture: Lateral recumbent
Angle: Oblique puncture
Direction: Toward intercostal space
Depth: 5-10 mm
Indications: Full sensation in chest, tuberculosis of lymph nobe

15. Epigastric Region

Point: Shuifen
Meridian: RN 9
Location: On anterior midline, 1 *cun* above umbilicus
Posture: Supine
Angle: Perpendicular puncture
Direction: Toward abdominal cavity
Depth: 15-30 mm
Indications: Ascites, abdominalgia, edema

Point: Xiawan
Meridian: RN 10
Location: On anterior midline, 2 *cun* above umbilicus
Posture: Supine
Angle: Perpendicular puncture
Direction: Toward abdominal cavity
Depth: 20-30 mm

Indications: Stomachalgia, vomiting, gastroptosis

Point: Jianli
Meridian: RN 11
Location: On anterior midline, 3 *cun* above umbilicus
Posture: Supine
Angle: Perpendicular puncture
Direction: Toward abdominal cavity
Depth: 15-30 mm
Indications: Stomachalgia, inappetence, gastroptosis

Point: Zhongwan
Meridian: RN 12
Location: On anterior midline, 4 *cun* above umbilicus
Posture: Supine
Angle: Perpendicular puncture
Direction: Toward abdominal cavity
Depth: 20-30 mm
Indications: Stomachalgia, gastric ulcer, gastritis

Point: Shangwan
Meridian: RN 13
Location: On anterior midline, 5 *cun* above umbilicus
Posture: Supine
Angle: Perpendicular puncture
Direction: Toward abdominal cavity
Depth: 20-30 mm
Indications: Stomachalgia, gastric ulcer, gastritis

Point: Juque
Meridian: RN 14
Location: On anterior midline, 6 *cun* above umbilicus
Posture: Supine
Angle: Perpendicular puncture
Direction: Toward thorax
Depth: 20-30 mm
Indications: Disorders of heart, vomiting, gastritis, manic-depressive psychosis

Point: Jiuwei
Meridian: RN 15
Location: On anterior midline, 1 *cun* below xiphisternal Ge
Posture: Supine
Angle: Perpendicular puncture
Direction: Toward thorax
Depth: 10-15 mm
Indications: Psychosis, angina pectoris, vomiting

Point: Shangqu
Meridian: KI 17
Location: 2 *cun* above umbilicus, 0.5 *cun* lateral to anterior midline
Posture: Supine
Angle: Perpendicular puncture
Direction: Toward abdominal cavity
Depth: 15-30 mm
Indications: Cholecystitis, duodenal ulcer, hepatitis

Point: Shiguan
Meridian: KI 18
Location: 3 *cun* above umbilicus, 0.5 *cun* lateral to anterior midline
Posture: Supine
Angle: Perpendicular puncture
Direction: Toward abdominal cavity
Depth: 15-30 mm
Indications: Cholecystitis, vomiting, coustipation, postpartum tormina

Point: Yindu
Meridian: KI 19
Location: 4 *cun* above umbilicus, 0.5 *cun* lateral to anterior midline
Posture: Supine
Angle: Perpendicular puncture
Direction: Toward abdominal cavity
Depth: 20-30 mm
Indications: Vomiting, diarrhea, abdominalgia

Point: Tonggu
Meridian: KI 20
Location: 5 *cun* above umbilicus, 0.5

cun lateral to anterior midline
Posture: Supine
Angle: Perpendicular puncture
Direction: Toward abdominal cavity
Depth: 20-30 mm
Indications: Vomiting, diarrhea, abdominalgia

Point: Youmen
Meridian: KI 21
Location: 6 *cun* above umbilicus, 0.5 *cun* lateral to anterior midline
Posture: Supine
Angle: Oblique puncture
Direction: Toward abdominal cavity
Depth: 20-30 mm
Indications: Vomiting, diarrhea, abdominalgia

Point: Burong
Meridian: SO 19
Location: 6 *cun* above umbilicus, 2 *cun* lateral to anterior midline
Posture: Supine
Angle: Oblique puncture
Direction: Toward abdominal cavity
Depth: 20-30 mm
Indications: Inappetence, gastric ulcer

Point: Chengman
Meridian: ST 20
Location: 5 *cun* above umbilicus, 2 *cun* lateral to anterior midline
Posture: Supine
Angle: Perpendicular puncture
Direction: Toward abdominal cavity
Depth: 15-30 mm
Indications: Inappetence, gastric ulcer, hepatic dysfunction

Point: Liangmen
Meridian: ST 21
Location: 4 *cun* above umbilicus, 2 *cun* lateral to anterior midline
Posture: Supine
Angle: Perpendicular puncture
Direction: Toward abdominal cavity

Depth: 15-30 mm
Indications: Gastritis, gastroneurosis, gastric ulcer

Point: Guanmen
Meridian: ST 22
Location: 3 *cun* above umbilicum, 2 *cun* lateral to anterior midline
Posture: Supine
Angle: Perpendicular puncture
Direction: Towards abdominal cavity
Depth: 15-30 mm
Indications: Gastroneurosis, gastric ulcer

Point: Taiyi
Meridian: ST 23
Location: 2 *cun* above umbilicus, 2 *cun* lateral to anterior midline
Posture: Supine
Angle: Perpendicular puncture
Direction: Toward abdominal cavity
Depth: 15-30 mm
Indications: Gastroneurosis, gastric ulcer

Point: Huaroumen
Meridian: ST 24
Location: 1 *cun* above umbilicus, 2 *cun* lateral to anterior midline
Posture: Supine
Angle: Perpendicular puncture
Direction: Toward abdominal cavity
Depth: 20-30 mm
Indications: Enteritis, manic-depressive psychosis, constipation

Point: Zhangmen
Meridian: LR 13
Location: On lateral side of abdomen, at lower border of free end of eleventh rib
Posture: Supine
Angle: Perpendicular puncture
Direction: Toward abdominal cavity
Depth: 15-20 mm
Indications: Pancreatitis, diabetes

Point: Qimen
Meridian: LR 14
Location: Directly below nipple, 4 *cun* lateral to anterior midline in sixth intercostal space
Posture: Supine
Angle: Oblique puncture
Direction: Toward abdominal cavity
Depth: 15-30 mm
Indications: Pleuritis, hepatitis, hepatic dysfunction

Point: Riyue
Meridian: GB 24
Location: Directly below nipple, 4 *cun* lateral to anterior midline in seventh intercostal space
Posture: Supine
Angle: Perpendicular puncture
Direction: Toward abdominal cavity
Depth: 20-30 mm
Indications: Cholecystitis, duodenal ulcer

Point: Fuai
Meridian: SP 16
Location: 3 *cun* above umbilicus, 4 *cun* lateral to anterior midline
Posture: Supine
Angle: Perpendicular puncture
Direction: Toward abdominal cavity
Depth: 15-30 mm
Indications: Dyspepsia, duodenal ulcer

16. Hypogastric Region

Point: Huiyin
Meridian: RN 1
Location: In perineum, between anus and posterior labial commissure in females and at root part of scrotum in males
Posture: Supine
Angle: Perpendicular puncture
Direction: Toward abdominal cavity
Depth: 15-30 mm

Indications: Anuresis, irregular menstruation, hysteroptosis, spermatorrhea

Point: Qugu
Meridian: RN 2
Location: On anterior midline at midpoint of superior border of the symphysis pubica
Posture: Supine
Angle: Perpendicular puncture
Direction: Toward abdominal cavity
Depth: 15-30 mm
Indications: Pelvic inflammation, urinary incontinence, spermatorrhea, impotence

Point: Zhongji
Meridian: RN 3
Location: On anterior midline, 4 *cun* below umbilicus
Posture: Supine
Angle: Perpendicular puncture
Direction: Toward abdominal cavity
Depth: 20-40 mm
Indications: Impotence, spermatorrhea, pelvic inflammation, irregular menstruation, leukorrhea

Point: Guanyuan
Meridian: RN 4
Location: On anterior midline, 3 *cun* below umbilicus
Posture: Supine
Angle: Perpendicular puncture
Direction: Toward abdominal cavity
Depth: 30-40 mm
Indications: Impotence, spermatorrhea, dysmenorrhea, irregular menstruation, keeping fit

Point: Shimen
Meridian: RN 5
Location: On anterior midline, 2 *cun* below umbilicus
Posture: Supine
Angle: Perpendicular puncture

Direction: Toward abdominal cavity
Depth: 15-30 mm
Indications: Difficulty in urination, gynecopathy

Point: Qihai
Meridian: RN 6
Location: On anterior midline, 1.5 *cun* below umbilicus
Posture: Supine
Angle: Perpendicular puncture
Direction: Toward abdominal cavity
Depth: 15-30 mm
Indications: Spermatorrhea, impotence, appendicitis, dysmenorrhea, enuresis, keeping fit

Point: Yinjiao
Meridian: RN 7
Location: On anterior midline, 1 *cun* below umbilicus
Posture: Supine
Angle: Perpendicular puncture
Direction: Toward abdominal cavity
Depth: 15-30 mm
Indications: Lumbago, peritonitis

Point: Shenque
Meridian: RN 8
Location: In center of umbilicus
Posture: Supine
Angle: Do not puncture with needle, salt moxibustion
Direction:
Depth:
Indications: Abdominal distension, diarrhea

Point: Daimai
Meridian: GB 26
Location: On lateral region of abdomen, 1.8 *cun* below Zhangmen (LR 13), directly below free end of eleventh rib and level with umbilicus
Posture: Lateral recumbent
Angle: Perpendicular puncture
Direction: Toward abdominal cavity

Depth: 15-25 mm
Indications: Irregular menstruation, hernia, leukorrhea

Point: Wushu
Meridian: GB 27
Location: On lateral region of abdomen, on anterior to anterior superior iliac spine and at level 3 *cun* below the umbilicus
Posture: Lateral recumbent
Angle: Perpendicular
Direction: Medially and inferiorly
Depth: 15-30 mm
Indications: Irregular menstruation, hernia, leukorrhea, lumbago

Point: Weidao
Meridian: GB 28
Location: On lateral region of abdomen, anterior and inferior to anterior superior iliac spine, 0.5 *cun* anterior and inferior to Wushu (GB 27)
Posture: Lateral recumbent
Angle: Oblique puncture
Direction: Medially and inferiorly
Depth: 15-30 mm
Indications: Hypogastralgia

Point: Juliao
Meridian: GB 29
Location: Midway between anterior superior iliac spine and highest point of greater trochanter of femur, on coxa
Posture: Lateral recumbent
Angle: Perpendicular puncture
Direction: Downward
Depth: 15-30 mm
Indications: Lumbocrural pain, paralysis

Point: Henggu
Meridian: KI 11
Location: 5 *cun* below umbilicus, 0.5 *cun* lateral to anterior midline
Posture: Supine

Angle: Perpendicular puncture
Direction: Toward abdominal cavity
Depth: 10-15 mm
Indications: Abdominalgia, dysentery, constipation

Point: Dahe
Meridian: KI 12
Location: 4 *cun* below umbilicus, 0.5 *cun* lateral to anterior midline
Posture: Supine
Angle: Perpendicular puncture
Direction: Toward abdominal cavity
Depth: 15-25 mm
Indications: Spermatorrhea, leukorrhea, cystitis

Point: Qixue
Meridian: KI 13
Location: 3 *cun* below umbilicus, 0.5 *cun* lateral to anterior midline
Posture: Supine
Angle: Perpendicular puncture
Direction: Toward abdominal cavity
Depth: 20-30 mm
Indications: Diarrhea, irregular menstruation, cystitis

Point: Siman
Meridian: KI 14
Location: 2 *cun* below umbilicus, 0.5 *cun* lateral to anterior midline
Posture: Supine
Angle: Perpendicular puncture
Direction: Toward abdominal cavity
Depth: 20-30 mm
Indications: Irregular menstruation, endometrorrhagia, postpartum tormina

Point: Zhongzhu
Meridian: KI 15
Location: 1 *cun* below umbilicus, 0.5 *cun* lateral to anterior midline
Posture: Supine
Angle: Perpendicular puncture
Direction: Toward abdominal cavity

Depth: 20-30 mm
Indications: Irregular menstruation, constipation, gastric ulcer
Point: Tianshu
Meridian: ST 25
Location: 2 *cun* lateral to center of umbilicus
Posture: Supine
Angle: Perpendicular puncture
Direction: Toward abdominal cavity
Depth: 20-30 mm
Indications: Abdominalgia, dysentery, constipation
Point: Wailing
Meridian: ST 26
Location: 1 *cun* lateral to anterior midline
Posture: Supine
Angle: Perpendicular puncture
Direction: Toward abdominal cavity
Depth: 15-30 mm
Indications: Abdominalgia, diarrhea
Point: Daju
Meridian: ST 27
Location: 2 *cun* below umbilicus, 2 *cun* lateral to anterior midline
Posture: Supine
Angle: Perpendicular puncture
Direction: Toward abdominal cavity
Depth: 15-30 mm
Indications: Distension of lower abdomen, hernia, spermatorrhea, prospermia
Point: Shuidao
Meridian: ST 28
Location: 3 *cun* below umbilicus, 2 *cun* lateral to anterior midline
Posture: Supine
Angle: Perpendicular puncture
Direction: Toward abdominal cavity
Depth: 15-30 mm
Indications: Hernia, anuresis
Point: Guilai

Meridian: ST 29
Location: 4 *cun* below umbilicus, 2 *cun* lateral to anterior midline
Posture: Supine
Angle: Perpendicular puncture
Direction: Toward abdominal cavity
Depth: 15-30 mm
Indications: Hernia, amenorrhea, hysteroptosis, cystitis
Point: Qichong
Meridian: ST 30
Location: Slightly superior to inguinal groove, 5 *cun* below umbilicus, 2 *cun* lateral to anterior midline
Posture: Supine
Angle: Perpendicular puncture
Direction: Medially and inferiorly
Depth: 10-15 mm
Indications: Irregular menstruation, peritonitis, ascites, hernia
Point: Chongmen
Meridian: SP 12
Location: On lateral side of inguinal groove, 3.5 *cun* above midpoint of upper border of symphysis pubica, lateral to external iliac artery
Posture: Supine
Angle: Oblique puncture
Direction: Medially and inferiorly
Depth: 15-30 mm
Indications: Orchitis, endometritis
Point: Fushe
Meridian: SP 13
Location: 4 *cun* below umbilicus, 0.7 *cun* above Chongmen (SP 12), 4 *cun* lateral to anterior midline
Posture: Supine
Angle: Perpendicular puncture
Direction: Toward pelvic cavity
Depth: 20-30 mm
Indications: Hernia, appendicitis, constipation
Point: Fujie

Meridian: SP 14
Location: 1.3 *cun* below Daheng (SP 15), 4 *cun* lateral to anterior midline
Posture: Supine
Angle: Perpendicular puncture
Direction: Toward abdominal cavity
Depth: 15-20 mm
Indications: Hernia, constipation, diarrhea

Point: Daheng
Meridian: SP 15
Location: 4 *cun* lateral to umbilicus
Posture: Supine
Angle: Perpendicular puncture
Direction: Toward abdominal cavity
Depth: 20-30 mm
Indications: Peritonitis, pyelonephrrtis, dysentery, constipation

Point: Jimai
Meridian: LR 12
Location: 2.5 *cun* lateral to anterior midline, lateral side of symphysis pubica, lateral and inferior to Qichong (ST 30) where femoral artery pulsates
Posture: Supine
Angle: Oblique puncture
Direction: Medially and inferiorly
Depth: 15-20 mm
Indications: Hernia

Point: Huangshu
Meridian: KI 16
Location: 0.5 *cun* lateral to umbilicus
Posture: Supine
Angle: Perpendicular puncture
Direction: Toward abdominal cavity
Depth: 20-30 mm
Indications: Gastritis, gastric ulcer, constipation

17. Upper Back

Point: Lingtai
Meridian: DU 10

Location: In midposterior line, in depression of inferior to spinous process of sixth thoracic vertebra
Posture: Sitting
Angle: Oblique puncture
Direction: Toward interspine
Depth: 5-10 mm
Indications: Bronchitis, asthma

Point: Shendao
Meridian: DU 11
Location: In midposterior line, on inferior to spinous process of fifth thoracic vertebra
Posture: Sitting
Angle: Oblique puncture
Direction: Toward interspine
Depth: 5-10 mm
Indications: Amnesia, hysteria, panic, spondylalgia

Point: Shenzhu
Meridian: DU 12
Location: In midposterior line, on inferior to spinous process of third thoracic vertebra
Posture: Sitting
Angle: Oblique puncture
Direction: Toward interspine
Depth: 5-10 mm
Indications: Chin cough, dyspepsia, pain along spinal column

Point: Taodao
Meridian: DU 13
Location: In midposterior line, on inferior to spinous process of first thoracic vertebra
Posture: Sitting
Angle: Oblique puncture
Direction: Toward interspine
Depth: 10 mm
Indications: Cold, headache, fever, epilepsy

Point: Dazhui
Meridian: DU 14

Location: In midposterior line, on inferior to spinous process of seventh cervical vertebra
Posture: Sitting
Angle: Oblique puncture
Direction: Toward interspine
Depth: 10 mm
Indications: Fever, schizophrenia, asthma, poliomyelitis

Point: Dazhu
Meridian: BL 11
Location: 1.5 *cun* lateral to lower border of spinous process of first thoracic vertebra
Posture: Sitting
Angle: Oblique puncture
Direction: Toward intercostal space
Depth: 10-15 mm
Indications: Cough, fever

Point: Fengmen
Meridian: BL 12
Location: 1.5 *cun* lateral to lower border of spinous process of second thoracic vertebra
Posture: Sitting
Angle: Oblique puncture
Direction: Toward intercostal space
Depth: 10-15 mm
Indications: Fever, cold, headache

Point: Feishu
Meridian: BL 13
Location: 1.5 *cun* lateral to lower border of spinous process of third thoracic vertebra
Posture: Sitting
Angle: Oblique puncture
Direction: Toward intercostal space
Depth: 10-15 mm
Indications: Disorders of the respiratory system

Point: Jueyinshu
Meridian: BL 14
Location: 1.5 *cun* lateral to lower bor-

der of spinous process of fourth thoracic vertebra
Posture: Sitting
Angle: Oblique puncture
Direction: Toward intercostal space
Depth: 10-15 mm
Indications: Cough, heart disorders, vomiting

Point: Xinshu
Meridian: BL 15
Location: 1.5 *cun* lateral to lower border of spinous process of fifth thoracic vertebra
Posture: Sitting
Angle: Oblique puncture
Direction: Toward intercostal space
Depth: 10-15 mm
Indications: Neurasthenia, insomnia, schizophrenia

Point: Dushu
Meridian: BL 16
Location: 1.5 *cun* lateral to lower border of spinous process of sixth thoracic vertebra
Posture: Sitting
Angle: Oblique puncture
Direction: Toward intercostal space
Depth: 10-15 mm
Indications: Heart disorders, abdominalgia

Point: Fufen
Meridian: BL 41
Location: 3 *cun* lateral to lower border of spinous process of second thoracic vertebra
Posture: Sitting
Angle: Oblique puncture
Direction: Toward intercostal space
Depth: 20-30 mm
Indications: Cold, stiffness of nape

Point: Pohu
Meridian: BL 42
Location: 3 *cun* lateral to lower border

of spinous process of third thoracic vertebra
Posture: Sitting
Angle: Oblique puncture
Direction: Toward intercostal space
Depth: 20-30 mm
Indications: Cough, asthma

Point: Gaohuang
Meridian: BL 43
Location: 3 *cun* lateral to lower border of spinous process of fourth thoracic vertebra
Posture: Sitting
Angle: Oblique puncture
Direction: Toward intercostal space
Depth: 15-20 mm
Indications: Asthma, neurasthenia

Point: Shentang
Meridian: BL 44
Location: 3 *cun* lateral to lower border of spinous process of fifth thoracic vertebra
Posture: Sitting
Angle: Oblique puncture
Direction: Toward intercostal space
Depth: 15-20 mm
Indications: Asthma, cough

Point: Yixi
Meridian: BL 45
Location: 3 *cun* lateral to lower border of spinous process of sixth thoracic vertebra
Posture: Sitting
Angle: Oblique puncture
Direction: Toward intercostal space
Depth: 10-15 mm
Indications: Asthma, cough, pain of shoulder and back

Point: Jianjing
Meridian: GB 21
Location: On shoulder, midway between Dazhui (GB 14) and acromion

Posture: Sitting
Angle: Perpendicular puncture
Direction: Toward thorax
Depth: 20-30 mm
Indications: Hypertension, mastitis, hypogalactia

Point: Tianliao
Meridian: SJ 15
Location: On scapular region, midway between Jianjing (GB 21) and Quyuan (SI 13) on superior angle of scapula
Posture: Sitting
Angle: Perpendicular puncture
Direction: Toward thorax
Depth: 10-20 mm
Indications: Stiffness of nape

Point: Naoshu
Meridian: SI 10
Location: On shoulder, inferior border of spine of scapula, directly above end of posterior axillary line
Posture: Sitting
Angle: Oblique puncture
Direction: Anteriorly
Depth: 15-25 mm
Indications: Pain in shoulder and arm

Point: Tianzong
Meridian: SI 11
Location: On scapular region, center of infraspinous fossa, level with fourth thoracic vertebra
Posture: Sitting
Angle: Oblique puncture
Direction: Slightly laterally
Depth: 10-15 mm
Indications: Scapulalgia

Point: Bingfeng
Meridian: SI 12
Location: On scapular region, center of supraspinous fossa, directly above Tianzong (SI 11). When arm lifted, point at site of depression

Posture: Sitting
Angle: Oblique puncture
Direction: Toward thorax
Indications: 10-15 mm
Depth: Cervicodynia, scapulalgia

Point: Quyuan
Meridian: SI 13
Location: On scapular region, medial extremity of supraspinous fossa, midway between Naoshu (SI 10) and spinous process of second thoracic vertebra
Posture: Sitting
Angle: Oblique puncture
Direction: Toward thorax
Depth: 15-25 mm
Indications: Cervicodynia, scapulalgia

Point: Jugu
Meridian: LI 16
Location: In upper aspect of shoulders, in depression between acromial extremity of clavicle and spine of scapular
Posture: Sitting
Angle: Perpendicular puncture
Direction: Toward shoulder joint
Depth: 8-10 mm
Indications: Scapulalgia

Point: Jianwaishu
Meridian: SI 14
Location: 3 *cun* lateral to lower border of spinous process of first thoracic vertebra
Posture: Sitting
Angle: Perpendicular puncture
Direction: Toward chest
Depth: 10-20 mm
Indications: Pain in shoulder and back

Point: Jianzhongshu
Meridian: SI 15
Location: 2 *cun* lateral to lower border of spinous process of seventh cervical vertebra

Posture: Sitting
Angle: Perpendicular puncture
Direction: Toward thorax
Depth: 10-20 mm
Indications: Cough, asthma

18. Median of Back

Point: Jizhong
Meridian: DU 6
Location: On midposterior line, in depression inferior to spinous process of eleventh thoracic vertebra
Posture: Prone
Angle: Perpendicular puncture
Direction: Toward interspine
Depth: 10-15 mm
Indications: Jaundice, hemorrhoids, epilepsy

Point: Zhongshu
Meridian: DU 7
Location: On midposterior line, in depression inferior to spinous process of tenth thoracic vertebra
Posture: Prone
Angle: Perpendicular puncture
Direction: Toward interspine
Depth: 10-15 mm
Indications: Esophagismus, lumbago

Point: Jinsuo
Meridian: DU 8
Location: On midposterior line, in depression inferior to spinous process of ninth thoracic vertebra
Posture: Prone
Angle: Perpendicular puncture
Direction: Toward interspine
Depth: 10-15 mm
Indications: Epilepsy, stomachalgia

Point: Zhiyang
Meridian: DU 9
Location: On midposterior line, in depression inferior to spinous process of seventh thoracic vertebra

Posture: Sitting
Angle: Oblique puncture
Direction: Toward interspine
Depth: 10-15 mm
Indications: Asthma, stomachalgia, rigid spine

Point: Geshu
Meridian: BL 17
Location: 1.5 *cun* lateral to lower border of spinous process of seventh thoracic vertebra
Posture: Sitting
Angle: Oblique puncture
Direction: Toward intercostal space
Depth: 15-20 mm
Indications: Gastritis, pleuritis, urticaria, vomiting

Point: Ganshu
Meridian: BL 18
Location: 1.5 *cun* lateral to lower border of spinous process of ninth thoracic vertebra
Posture: Prone
Angle: Perpendicular puncture
Direction: Toward intercostal space
Depth: 6-10 mm
Indications: Hepathopathy, gastropathy, ophthalmopathy, lethargy

Point: Danshu
Meridian: BL 19
Location: 1.5 *cun* lateral to lower border of spinous process of tenth thoracic vertebra
Posture: Prone
Angle: Perpendicular puncture
Direction: Toward intercostal space
Depth: 6-10 mm
Indications: Disorders of liver and gallbladder, lethargy, gastritis

Point: Pishu
Meridian: BL 20
Location: 1.5 *cun* lateral to lower border of spinous process of eleventh

thoracic vertebra
Posture: Prone
Angle: Perpendicular puncture
Direction: Toward intercostal space
Depth: 6-10 mm
Indications: Disorders of digestive system, hematopathy

Point: Weishu
Meridian: BL 21
Location: 1.5 *cun* lateral to lower border of spinous process of twelfth thoracic vertebra
Posture: Prone
Angle: Perpendicular puncture
Direction: Toward thorax
Depth: 15-20 mm
Indications: Disorders of digestive system

Point: Geguan
Meridian: BL 46
Location: 3 *cun* lateral to lower border of spinous process of seventh thoracic vertebra
Posture: Sitting
Angle: Oblique puncture
Direction: Toward intercostal space
Depth: 10-15 mm
Indications: Inappetence, pain in shoulder and back

Point: Hunmen
Meridian: BL 47
Location: 3 *cun* lateral to lower border of spinous process of ninth thoracic vertebra
Posture: Prone
Angle: Perpendicular puncture
Direction: Toward intercostal space
Depth: 10-15 mm
Indications: Disorders of liver and pancreas

Point: Yanggang
Meridian: BL 48
Location: 3 *cun* lateral to lower border

of spinous process of tenth thoracic vertebra
Posture: Prone
Angle: Perpendicular puncture
Direction: Toward intercostal space
Depth: 10-15 mm
Indications: Diarrhea, jaundice

Point: Yishe
Meridian: BL 49
Location: 3 *cun* lateral to lower border of spinous process of eleventh thoracic vertebra
Posture: Prone
Angle: Perpendicular puncture
Direction: Toward intercostal space
Depth: 10-15 mm
Indications: Diarrhea, jaundice, inappetence

Point: Weicang
Meridian: BL 50
Location: 3 *cun* lateral lower border of spinous process of twelfth thoracic vertebra
Posture: Prone
Angle: Perpendicular puncture
Direction: Toward thorax
Depth: 10-15 mm
Indications: Disorders of stomach and duodenum

19. Lower Back

Point: Changqiang
Meridian: DU 1
Location: Midway between tip of coccyx and anus
Posture: Prone
Angle: Oblique puncture
Direction: Slightly medially
Depth: 15-30 mm
Indications: Hemorrhoids, spermatorrhea, proctoptosis

Point: Yaoshu
Meridian: DU 2
Location: On midposterior line and sacrum, at sacral hiatus
Posture: Prone
Angle: Oblique puncture
Direction: Upward
Depth: 10-15 mm
Indications: Hemorrhoids, irregular menstruation, lumbago, enteritis

Point: Yaoyangguan
Meridian: DU 3
Location: On lumbar region and midposterior line, inferior to spinous process of fourth lumbar vertebra
Posture: Prone
Angle: Perpendicular puncture
Direction: Toward spinous process
Depth: 8-10 mm
Indications: Impotence, spermatorrhea, irregular menstruation, lumbago

Point: Mingmen
Meridian: DU 4
Location: On lumbar region and midposterior line, inferior to spinous process of second lumbar vertebra
Posture: Prone
Angle: Perpendicular puncture
Direction: Toward spinous process
Depth: 8-10 mm
Indications: Impotence, spermatorrhea, leukorrhea, lumbago

Point: Xuanshu
Meridian: DU 5
Location: On lumbar region and midposterior line, inferior to spinous process of first lumbar vertebra
Posture: Prone
Angle: Perpendicular puncture
Direction: Toward spinous process
Depth: 8-10 mm
Indications: Dyspepsia, diarrhea

Point: Sanjiaoshu
Meridian: BL 22

Location: On lumbar region, 1.5 *cun* lateral to lower border of spinous process of first lumbar vertebra
Posture: Prone
Angle: Perpendicular puncture
Direction: Toward abdomen
Depth: 15-20 mm
Indications: Diarrhea, edema, pain along spinal column

Point: Shenshu
Meridian: BL 23
Location: On lumbar region, 1.5 *cun* lateral to lower border of spinous process of second lumbar vertebra
Posture: Prone
Angle: Perpendicular puncture
Direction: Toward abdomen
Depth: 10-20 mm
Indications: Spermatorrhea, enuresis, impotence, dizziness, irregular menstruation

Point: Qihaishu
Meridian: BL 24
Location: On lumbar region, 1.5 *cun* lateral to lower border of spinous process of third lumbar vertebra
Posture: Prone
Angle: Perpendicular puncture
Direction: Toward abdomen
Depth: 15-20 mm
Indications: Lumbago

Point: Dachangshu
Meridian: BL 25
Location: On lumbar region, 1.5 *cun* lateral to lower border of spinous process of fourth lumbar vertebra
Posture: Prone
Angle: Perpendicular puncture
Direction: Toward pelvis
Depth: 20-30 mm
Indications: Lumbago, dysentery, diarrhea

Point: Guanyuanshu

Meridian: BL 26
Location: On lumbar region, 1.5 *cun* lateral to lower border of spinous process of fifth lumbar vertebra
Posture: Prone
Angle: Perpendicular puncture
Direction: Toward pelvis
Depth: 20-30 mm
Indications: Lumbago, disorders of genitourinary system

Point: Xiaochangshu
Meridian: BL 27
Location: On sacrum, level with first posterior sacral foramen, 1.5 *cun* lateral to median sacral crest
Posture: Prone
Angle: Perpendicular puncture
Direction: Toward pelvis
Depth: 20-30 mm
Indications: Lumbago, disorders of genitourinary system

Point: Pangguangshu
Meridian: BL 28
Location: 1.5 *cun* lateral to lower border of spinous process of fourth thoracic vertebra
Posture: Prone
Angle: Perpendicular puncture
Direction: Toward pelvis
Depth: 20-30 mm
Indications: Lumbago, disorders of genitourinary system

Point: Zhonglushu
Meridian: BL 29
Location: On sacrum, level with third posterior sacral foramen, 1.5 *cun* lateral to median sacral crest
Posture: Prone
Angle: Perpendicular puncture
Direction: Toward pelvis
Depth: 15-30 mm
Indications: Dysentery, hernia, intestinal hemorrhage

Point: Baihuanshu
Meridian: BL 30
Location: On sacrum, level with fourth posterior sacral foramen, 1.5 *cun* lateral to median sacral crest
Posture: Prone
Angle: Perpendicular puncture
Direction: Toward pelvis
Depth: 15-30 mm
Indications: Spermatorrhea, irregular menstruation, enteritis

Point: Shangliao
Meridian: BL 31
Location: On sacrum, level with first posterior sacral foramen, between posterior superior iliac spine and midposterior line
Posture: Prone
Angle: Perpendicular puncture
Direction: Toward foramen
Depth: 15-30 mm
Indications: Sciatica, disorders of genitourinary system

Point: Ciliao
Meridian: BL 32
Location: On sacrum, level with second posterior sacral foramen, at medial and inferior to posterior superior iliac spine
Posture: Prone
Angle: Perpendicular puncture
Direction: Toward foramen
Depth: 15-30 mm
Indications: Sciatica, disorders of genitourinary system

Point: Zhongliao
Meridian: BL 33
Location: On sacrum, level with third posterior sacral foramen, at medial and inferior to Ciliao (BL 32)
Posture: Prone
Angle: Perpendicular puncture
Direction: Toward foramen

Depth: 15-30 mm
Indications: Sciatica, disorders of genitourinary system

Point: Xialiao
Meridian: BL 34
Location: On sacrum, level with fourth posterior sacral foramen, at medial and inferior to Zhongliao (BL 33)
Posture: Prone
Angle: Perpendicular puncture
Direction: Toward foramen
Depth: 15-30 mm
Indications: Sciatica, disorders of genitourinary system

Point: Huiyang
Meridian: BL 35
Location: On sacrum, 0.5 *cun* lateral to lower end of coccyx
Posture: Prone
Angle: Perpendicular puncture
Direction: Toward mates
Depth: 15-20 mm
Indications: Impotence, dysentery, hematochezia, diarrhea

Point: Huangmen
Meridian: BL 51
Location: On lumbus, 3 *cun* lateral to lower border of spinous process of first lumbar vertebra
Posture: Prone
Angle: Perpendicular puncture
Direction: Toward abdomen
Depth: 15-30 mm
Indications: Disorders of stomach and duodenum

Point: Zhishi
Meridian: BL 52
Location: On lumbus, 3 *cun* lateral to lower border of spinous process of second lumbar vertebra
Posture: Prone
Angle: Perpendicular puncture
Direction: Toward umbilicus

Depth: 20-30 mm

Indications: Spermatorrhea, impotence, dedma, difficult micturition

Point: Baohuang

Meridian: BL 53

Location: On mates, level with second posterior sacral foramen, 3 *cun* lateral to median sacral crest

Posture: Prone

Angle: Perpendicular puncture

Direction: Toward pelvis

Depth: 20-30 mm

Indications: Anuresis, abdominal distension

Point: Zhibian

Meridian: BL 54

Location: On sacrum, level with fourth posterior sacral foramen, 3 *cun* lateral to median sacral crest

Posture: Prone

Angle: Perpendicular puncture

Direction: Toward pelvis

Depth: 20-30 mm

Indications: Anuresis, sciatica, dysentery

Point: Jingmen

Meridian: GB 25

Location: On lateral region of lumbus, 1.8 *cun* posterior to Zhangmen (LR 13), on lower border of free end of twelfth rib

Posture: Prone

Angle: Perpendicular puncture

Direction: Toward pelvis

Depth: 10-20 mm

Indications: Anuresis, sciatica, abdominal distension, pain in waist and hypochondrium

20. Anterior of Thigh

Point: Biguan

Meridian: ST 31

Location: On line joining anterior superior iliac spine and base of patella, in depression on lateral side of sartorius muscle. When thigh flexed, in a line level with perineum

Posture: Sitting

Angle: Perpendicular puncture

Direction: Posteriorly

Depth: 20-30 mm

Indications: Poliomyelitis, hemiparalysis

Point: Futu

Meridian: ST 32

Location: On line joining anterior superior iliac spine and base of patella, 6 *cun* above base of patella

Posture: Supine

Angle: Perpendicular puncture

Direction: Posteriorly

Depth: 20-30 mm

Indications: Paralysis or dyskinesia of lower limb

Point: Yinshi

Meridian: ST 33

Location: On line joining anterior superior iliac spine and base of patella, 3 *cun* above base of patella

Posture: Supine

Angle: Perpendicular puncture

Direction: Posteriorly

Depth: 15-20 mm

Indications: Paralysis, dyskinesia of lower limb

Point: Liangqiu

Meridian: ST 34

Location: When knee flexed, on line joining anterior superior iliac spine and base of patella, 2 *cun* above base of patella

Posture: Supine

Angle: Oblique puncture

Direction: Toward internal

Depth: 15-20 mm

Indications: Paralysis of lower limb,

stomachalgia, mastitis

21. Antero-Medinal of Thigh

Point: Xuehai
Meridian: SP 10
Location: When knee flexed, 2 *cun* above medial end of base of patella, on bulge of medial end of quadruceps muscle of thigh
Posture: Supine
Angle: Perpendicular puncture
Direction: Posterior
Depth: 20-30 mm
Indications: Subintrant, menstruation, urticaria, neurodermatitis

Point: Jimen
Meridian: SP 11
Location: 6 *cun* above Xuehai (SP 10), on line drawn from Xuehai to Chongmen (SP 12)
Posture: Supine
Angle: Perpendicular puncture
Direction: Laterally
Depth: 15-20 mm
Indications: Anuresis, spermatorrhea, proctoptosis

Point: Ququan
Meridian: LR 8
Location: When knee flexed, on anterior border of insertion of semimembranosus muscle and semitendinosus muscle, at medial end of genual crease and posterior border of internal epicondyle of femur
Posture: Supine
Angle: Perpendicular puncture
Direction: Toward joint
Depth: 8-10 mm
Indications: Impotence, spermatorrhea, hernia

Point: Yinbao
Meridian: LR 9
Location: 4 *cun* above medial epicondyle of femur, between vastus medialis and sartorius muscles
Posture: Supine
Angle: Perpendicular puncture
Direction: Laterally
Depth: 15-20 mm
Indications: Irregular menstruation, difficult micturition

Point: Zuwuli
Meridian: LR 10
Location: 3 *cun* directly below Qichong (ST 30) on lateral border of long abductor muscle, and on lower border of public tubercle
Posture: Supine
Angle: Perpendicular puncture
Direction: Laterally
Depth: 15-20 mm
Indications: Abdominal distension, anuresis

Point: Yinlian
Meridian: LR 11
Location: 2 *cun* directly below Qichong (ST 30) on lateral border of long abductor muscle, and on lower border of public tubercle
Posture: Supine
Angle: Perpendicular puncture
Direction: Laterally
Depth: 15-20 mm
Indications: Irregular menstruation, cystitis

22. Anterior of Leg

Point: Dubi
Meridian: ST 35
Location: On knee, when knee flexed, point in depression lateral to patella and patella ligament
Posture: Supine
Angle: Oblique puncture
Direction: Toward joint
Depth: 15-20 mm

Indications: Disorders of joint

Point: Zusanli
Meridian: ST 36
Location: 3 *cun* below Dubi (ST 35), a finger-breadth (middle finger) lateral to anterior crest of tibia
Posture: Supine
Angle: Perpendicular puncture
Direction: Posteriorly
Depth: 20-30 mm
Indications: Stomachalgia, hypertension, paralysis of lower limb, neurasthenia, keeping fit

Point: Shangjuxu
Meridian: ST 37
Location: 6 *cun* below Dubi (ST 35), a finger-breadth (middle finger) lateral to anterior crest of tibia
Posture: Supine
Angle: Perpendicular puncture
Direction: Posteriorly
Depth: 20-30 mm
Indications: Appendicitis, dysentery, paralysis of lower limb

Point: Tiaokou
Meridian: ST 38
Location: 8 *cun* below Dubi (ST 35), a finger-breadth (middle finger) lateral to anterior crest of tibis
Posture: Supine
Angle: Perpendicular puncture
Direction: Posteriorly
Depth: 15-20 mm
Indications: Numbness of leg, hypogatralgia

Point: Xiajuxu
Meridian: ST 39
Location: 9 *cun* below Dubi (ST 35), a finger-breadth (middle finger) lateral to anterior crest of tibia
Posture: Supine
Angle: Perpendicular puncture
Direction: Posteriorly

Depth: 15-20 mm
Indications: Hemiparalysis, abdominalgia

Point: Fenglong
Meridian: ST 40
Location: 8 *cun* above most prominent part of lateral malleolus, 2 finger-breadth (middle finger) lateral to anterior crest of tibia
Posture: Supine
Angle: Perpendicular puncture
Direction: Posteriorly
Depth: 15-20 mm
Indications: Enteritis, dizziness, cough, asthma

23. Antero-Medial of Leg

Point: Sanyinjiao
Meridian: SP 6
Location: 3 *cun* above most prominent part of medial malleolus, posterior to medial border of tibia
Posture: Supine
Angle: Oblique puncture
Direction: Laterally
Depth: 10-15 mm
Indications: Genitourinary disorders, hypertension, insomnia, eczema

Point: Lougu
Meridian: SP 7
Location: 6 *cun* above most prominent part of medial malleolus, on line drawn from most prominent part of medial malleolus to Yinglingquan (SP 9), posterior to medial border of tibia
Posture: Supine
Angle: Perpendicular puncture
Direction: Laterally
Depth: 10-15 mm
Indications: Gynecopathy, abdominal distension, enteritis

Point: Diji

Meridian: SP 8

Location: 3 *cun* below Yinlingquan (SP 9), on line drawn from most prominent part of medial malleolus to Yinlingquan (SP 9)

Posture: Supine

Angle: Perpendicular puncture

Direction: Laterally

Depth: 10-15 mm

Indications: Gynecopathy, inappentence

Point: Yinlingquan

Meridian: SP 9

Location: In depression on posteroinferior to medial condyle of tibia

Posture: Supine

Angle: Perpendicular puncture

Direction: Upwards

Depth: 15-20 mm

Indications: Irregular menstruation, abdominal distension, lumbago

Point: Ligou

Meridian: LR 5

Location: 5 *cun* above most prominent part of medial malleolus, on center of medial aspect of tibia

Posture: Supine

Angle: Oblique puncture

Direction: Downward

Depth: 10-15 mm

Indications: Disorders of female reproductive system, anuresis, spermatorrhea, urticaria

Point: Zhongdu

Meridian: LR 6

Location: 6 *cun* above most prominent part of medial malleolus, on center of medial aspect of tibia

Posture: Supine

Angle: Oblique puncture

Direction: Downward

Depth: 10-15 mm

Indications: Endometrorrhagia, hernia, hypogastralgia

Point: Xiguan

Meridian: LR 7

Location: Posteroinferior to medial condyle of tibia and 1 *cun* posterior to Yinlingquan (SP 9), in upper portion of medial head of gastrocnemius muscle

Posture: Supine

Angle: Oblique puncture

Direction: Toward joint

Depth: 8-10 mm

Indications: Gonitis

Point: Taixi

Meridian: KI 3

Location: On medial region of foot, posterior to medial malleolus, between most prominent part of medial malleolus and Achille's tendon

Posture: Supine

Angle: Oblique puncture

Direction: Laterally

Depth: 8-10 mm

Indications: Neurasthemia, toothache, lumbago, nephropathy

Point: Dazhong

Meridian: KI 4

Location: On medial region of foot posterior to medial malleolus, anterior to medial side, of attachment of Achille's tendon

Posture: Supine

Angle: Oblique puncture

Direction: Laterally

Depth: 8-10 mm

Indications: Tonsillitis, hemoptysis, dementia, somnolence

Point: Fuliu

Meridian: KI 7

Location: On medial region of leg, 2 *cun* directly above Taixi (KI 3), anterior to Achille's tendon

Posture: Supine

Angle: Oblique puncture
Direction: Downward
Depth: 10-15 mm
Indications: Heart failure, night sweats, disorders of genitourary system

Point: Jiaoxin
Meridian: KI 8
Location: 2 *cun* directly above Taixi (KI 3), 0.5 *cun* anterior to Fuliu (KI 7), posterior to medial border of tibia
Posture: Supine
Angle: Perpendicular puncture
Direction: Downward
Depth: 8-10 mm
Indications: Irregular menstruation, heart failure, constipation

Point: Zhubin
Meridian: KI 9
Location: On line drawn from Taixi (KI 3) to Yingu (KI 10), 5 *cun* above Taixi
Posture: Supine
Angle: Perpendicular puncture
Direction: Laterally
Depth: 8-10 mm
Indications: Detoxication, systremma, manic-depressive psychosis

Point: Yingu
Meridian: KI 10
Location: On medial side of popliteal fossa, between tendons of semitendinosus and semimembranosus muscles when knee flexed
Posture: Supine
Angle: Perpendicular puncture
Direction: Laterally
Depth: 8-10 mm
Indications: Disorders of reproductive system, hypogastralgia

24. Anterior of Foot

Point: Jiexi

Meridian: ST 41
Location: At center of crease of junction of dorsum of foot and leg, between tendons of long extensor muscles of great toe and toe
Posture: Supine
Angle: Oblique puncture
Direction: Medially
Depth: 10-20 mm
Indications: Headache, paralysis of lower limb, palsy of eyelid

Point: Chongyang
Meridian: ST 42
Location: At highest point of dorsum of foot, between tendons of long extensor muscles of great toe and long extensor muscle of toe, where dorsal artery of foot is palpable
Posture: Supine
Angle: Oblique puncture
Direction: Toward sole
Depth: 8-10 mm
Indications: Toothache, inappentence, paralysis of lower limb

Point: Xiangu
Meridian: ST 43
Location: In depression distal to junction of second and third metataral bones
Posture: Supine
Angle: Oblique puncture
Direction: Toward sole
Depth: 8-10 mm
Indications: Mastitis, headache

Point: Neiting
Meridian: ST 44
Location: Proximal to web margin between second and third toes
Posture: Supine
Angle: Oblique puncture
Direction: Toward sole
Depth: 8-10 mm
Indications: Stomachalgia, toothache,

headache, insomnia, tonsillitis

Point: Lidui
Meridian: ST 45
Location: On lateral side of second toe, 0.1 *cun* proximal to corner of nail
Posture: Supine
Angle: Oblique puncture
Direction: Toward heel
Depth: 5 mm
Indications: Hysteria, dyspepsia, cerebral hemorrhage, insomnia, tonsillitis

25. Medial Region of Foot

Point: Dadun
Meridian: LR 1
Location: On lateral side of dorsum of terminal phalanx of big toe, 0.1 *cun* proximal to lateral proximal corner of nail
Posture: Supine
Angle: Oblique puncture
Direction: Toward sole
Depth: 5 mm
Indications: Enuresis, profuse menstruation, hysteroptosis, orchitis

Point: Xingjian
Meridian: LR 2
Location: On dorsum foot, between first and second toes, proximal to margin of web
Posture: Supine
Angle: Oblique puncture
Direction: Toward sole
Depth: 8-10 mm
Indications: Cholelithiasis, coma, headache, insomnia, anuresis

Point: Taichong
Meridian: LR 3
Location: On dorsum of foot, at depression of posterior end of first interosseous metatarsal space
Posture: Supine

Angle: Perpendicular puncture
Direction: Toward sole
Depth: 8-10 mm
Indications: Headache, endometrorrhagia, mastitis, eye disorders

Point: Zhongfeng
Meridian: LR 4
Location: On dorsum of foot, anterior to medial malleolus, on line joining Shangqiu (SP 5) and Jiexi (ST 41), medial to tendon of anterior tibial muscle
Posture: Supine
Angle: Oblique puncture
Direction: Toward joint
Depth: 8-10 mm
Indications: Spermatorrhea, anuresis, hernia, lumbago

Point: Yinbai
Meridian: SP 1
Location: On medial side of big toe, 0.1 *cun* proximal to corner of nail
Posture: Supine
Angle: Oblique puncture
Direction: Laterally
Depth: 5 mm
Indications: Irregular menstruation, endometrorrhagia, dreaminess, manic-depressive psychosis

Point: Dadu
Meridian: SP 2
Location: On medial side of big toe, distal and inferior to first metatarsal phalangeal joint
Posture: Supine
Angle: Oblique puncture
Direction: Laterally
Depth: 8-10 mm
Indications: Diabetes, fever, stomachalgia, lasstitude

Point: Taibai
Meridian: SP 3
Location: On medial side of big toe,

proximal and inferior to first metatarsal phalangeal joint
Posture: Supine
Angle: Oblique puncture
Direction: Laterally
Depth: 8-10 mm
Indications: Diabetes, stomachalgia, lassitude, fever

Point: Gongsun
Meridian: SP 4
Location: On medial side of big toe, distal and inferior to base of first metatarsal bone
Posture: Supine
Angle: Oblique puncture
Direction: Laterally
Depth: 8-10 mm
Indications: Vomiting, inappentence

Point: Shangqiu
Meridian: SP 5
Location: In depression distal and inferior to medial malleolus, midway between tip of medial malleolus and tubercle of scaphoid bone
Posture: Supine
Angle: Oblique puncture
Direction: Toward joint
Depth: 8-10 mm
Indications: Lassitude, stiff tongue, abdominal distension

Point: Yongquan
Meridian: KI 1
Location: At junction of anterior and middle 1/3 of sole
Posture: Supine
Angle: Perpendicular puncture
Direction: Toward dorsum of foot
Depth: 10-15 mm
Indications: Shock, heliosis, nephritis, edema

Point: Rangu
Meridian: KI 2
Location: On medial border of foot,

inferior to tuberosity of navicular bone
Posture: Supine
Angle: Perpendicular puncture
Direction: Laterally
Depth: 8-10 mm
Indications: Otitis media, irregular menstruation, diabetes

Point: Shuiquan
Meridian: KI 5
Location: Posteroinferior to medial malleolus, 1 *cun* directly below Taixi (KI 3), medial side of tuberosity of calcaneum
Posture: Supine
Angle: Oblique puncture
Direction: Laterally
Depth: 8-10 mm
Indications: Gynecopathy, disorders of urinary system

Point: Zhaohai
Meridian: KI 6
Location: Inferior to tip of medial malleolus
Posture: Supine
Angle: Perpendicular puncture
Direction: Laterally
Depth: 8-10 mm
Indications: Gynecopathy, sore throat, forequent micturition

26. Posterior of Thigh

Point: Chengfu
Meridian: BL 36
Location: In middle of transverse gluteal fold
Posture: Prone
Angle: Perpendicular puncture
Direction: Anteriorly
Depth: 30-60 mm
Indications: Sciatica, paralysis of lower limb

Point: Yinmen

Meridian: BL 37
Location: 6 *cun* below Chengfu (BL 36), on line joining Chengfu and Weizhong (BL 40)
Posture: Prone
Angle: Perpendicular puncture
Direction: 30-50 mm
Depth: Sciatica, paralysis of lower limb

Point: Fuxi
Meridian: BL 38
Location: Lateral end of transverse crease of popliteal fossa, 1 *cun* above Weiyang (BL 39), on medial side of tendon of biceps muscle of thigh
Posture: Prone
Angle: Oblique puncture
Direction: Anteriorly
Depth: 15-20 mm
Indications: Sciatica, paralysis of lower limb

27. Lateral of Thigh

Point: Huantiao
Meridian: GB 30
Location: At junction of middle and lateral 1/3 of distance between highest point of great trochanter of thigh and sacral hiatus
Posture: Prone
Angle: Perpendicular puncture
Direction: Anteriorly
Depth: 40-60 mm
Indications: Sciatica, paralysis of lower limb

Point: Fengshi
Meridian: GB 31
Location: On midline of lateral aspect of thigh, 7 *cun* above transverse popliteal crease. When patient stands erect with hands close at sides, where tip of middle finger touches in normal-proportioned person
Posture: Lateral recumbent
Angle: Perpendicular puncture
Direction: Medially
Depth: 20-40 mm
Indications: Hemiparalysis, palsy of lower limb, spasm

Point: Zhongdu
Meridian: GB 32
Location: 2 *cun* below Fengshi, 5 *cun* above transverse popliteal crease, between musculus vastus lateralis and biceps muscle of thigh
Posture: Lateral recumbent
Angle: Perpendicular puncture
Direction: Medially
Depth: 10-20 mm
Indications: Hemiparalysis

Point: Xiyangguan
Meridian: GB 33
Location: Lateral to knee, 3 *cun* above Yanglingquan (GB 34), superior to external epicondyle of femur
Posture: Prone
Angle: Perpendicular puncture
Direction: Medially
Depth: 10-20 mm
Indications: Numbness of leg

28. Posterior of Leg

Point: Weiyang
Meridian: BL 39
Location: At lateral end of transverse popliteal fold, on medial border of tendon of biceps muscle of thigh
Posture: Prone
Angle: Perpendicular puncture
Direction: Anteriorly
Depth: 10-20 mm
Indications: Stiffness along spinal column

Point: Weizhong
Meridian: BL 40

Location: Midpoint at transverse crease of popliteal fossa, between tendons of biceps muscle of thigh and semitendiness muscle
Posture: Prone
Angle: Perpendicular puncture
Direction: Anteriorly
Depth: 10-20 mm
Indications: Paralysis of lower limb, heliosis, lumbago

Point: Heyang
Meridian: BL 55
Location: On line joining Weiyang (BL 40) and Chengshan (BL 57), 2 *cun* below Weizhong
Posture: Prone
Angle: Perpendicular puncture
Direction: Anteriorly
Depth: 15-30 mm
Indications: Weakness of lower limb, sciatica

Point: Chengjin
Meridian: BL 56
Location: On line joining Weizhong (BL 40) and Chengshan (BL 57), in center of belly of gastrocnemius muscle, 5 *cun* below Weizhong
Posture: Prone
Angle: Perpendicular puncture
Direction: Anteriorly
Depth: 15-30 mm
Indications: Weakness of lower limb, sciatica

Point: Chengshan
Meridian: BL 57
Location: On center of posterior region of leg, between Weizhong (BL 40) and Kunlun (BL 60), lower border of belly of gastrocnemius muscle
Posture: Prone
Angle: Perpendicular puncture
Direction: Anteriorly

Depth: 15-25 mm
Indications: Lassitude of lower limb, sciatica, hemorrhoids, constipation

Point: Feiyang
Meridian: BL 58
Location: Posterior to lateral malleolus, 7 *cun* directly above Kunlun (BL 60), 1 *cun* inferior and lateral to Chengshan (BL 57)
Posture: Prone
Angle: Perpendicular puncture
Direction: Anteriorly
Depth: 15-25 mm
Indications: Headache, nasal obstruction, lumbago, lassitude of lower limb

Point: Fuyang
Meridian: BL 59
Location: Posterior to lateral malleolus, 3 *cun* directly above Kunlun (BL 60)
Posture: Prone
Angle: Perpendicular puncture
Direction: Anteriorly
Depth: 10-20 mm
Indications: Sciatica, lassitude of lower limb

29. Lateral Region of Leg

Point: Yanglingquan
Meridian: GB 34
Location: Anterior and inferior to head of fibula
Posture: Prone
Angle: Perpendicular puncture
Direction: Medially
Depth: 10-15 mm
Indications: Prosopalgia, headache, hemiparalysis, disorders of biliary tract

Point: Yangjiao
Meridian: GB 35
Location: 7 *cun* above tip of lateral

malleolus, on posterior border of fibula

Posture: Prone

Angle: Perpendicular puncture

Direction: Medially

Depth: 10-20 mm

Indications: Pain and fullness in chest and hypochondrium, sciatica

Point: Waiqiu

Meridian: GB 36

Location: 7 *cun* above tip of lateral malleolus, on anterior border of fibula

Posture: Prone

Angle: Perpendicular puncture

Direction: Medially

Depth: 10-20 mm

Indications: Sciatica

Point: Guangming

Meridian: GB 37

Location: 5 *cun* above tip of lateral malleolus, on anterior border of fibula

Posture: Prone

Angle: Perpendicular puncture

Direction: Medially

Depth: 15-20 mm

Indications: Mastitis, eye disorders, pain of lower limb

Point: Yangfu

Meridian: GB 38

Location: 4 *cun* above tip of lateral malleolus, slightly anterior to anterior border of fibula

Posture: Prone

Angle: Perpendicular puncture

Direction: Medially

Depth: 10-15 mm

Indications: Migraine, sciatica

Point: Xuanzhong

Meridian: GB 39

Location: 3 *cun* above tip of lateral malleolus, on anterior border of fib-ula

Posture: Prone

Angle: Perpendular puncture

Direction: Medially

Depth: 10-15 mm

Indications: Paralysis of lower limb, stiff neck, blood stasis

30. Posterior and Lateral Region of Foot

Point: Kunlun

Meridian: BL 60

Location: Posterior to lateral malleolus between most prominent part of external malleolus and Achilles' tendon

Posture: Prone

Angle: Perpendicular puncture

Direction: Medially

Depth: 8-10 mm

Indications: Paralysis of lower limb, headache, dysentery

Point: Pucan

Meridian: BL 61

Location: Posterior and inferior to external malleolus, directly below Kunlun (BL 60), lateral side to calcameus

Posture: Prone

Angle: Oblique puncture

Direction: Toward joint

Depth: 5 mm

Indications: Lumbago, painful heels

Point: Shenmai

Meridian: BL 62

Location: In depression directly below external malleolus

Posture: Prone

Angle: Oblique puncture

Direction: Toward joint

Depth: 5 mm

Indications: Headache, dizziness, epilepsy

Point: Jinmen
Meridian: BL 63
Location: Directly below anterior border of external malleolus, inferior border of cuboid bone
Posture: Prone
Angle: Oblique puncture
Direction: Toward joint
Depth: 5 mm
Indications: Infantile convulsion, palsy of lower limb

Point: Jinggu
Meridian: BL 64
Location: Inferior to tuberosity of fifth metatarsal bone
Posture: Prone
Angle: Oblique puncture
Direction: Medially
Depth: 5-10 mm
Indications: Hypertension, headache, dizziness

Point: Shugu
Meridian: BL 65
Location: Proximal to fifth metatarsophalangeal joint
Posture: Prone
Angle: Oblique puncture
Direction: Medially
Depth: 5-10 mm
Indications: Hypertension, headache, dizziness

Point: Zutonggu
Meridian: BL 66
Location: Distal to fifth metatarsophalangeal joint
Posture: Supine
Angle: Oblique puncture
Direction: Medially
Depth: 5 mm
Indications: Cerebral hemorrhage, headache, dizziness

Point: Zhiyin
Meridian: BL 67

Location: On lateral side of small toe, 0.1 *cun* proximal to corner of nail
Posture: Supine
Angle: Oblique puncture
Direction: Toward root
Depth: 5 mm
Indications: Difficult labor, correction for position of fetus

Point: Qiuxu
Meridian: GB 40
Location: Anterior and inferior to external malleolus, on lateral side of tendon of long extensor muscle of toe
Posture: Supine
Angle: Perpendicular puncture
Direction: Toward joint
Depth: 8-10 mm
Indications: Pain in liver and sleen regions

Point: Zhulinqi
Meridian: GB 41
Location: On lateral side of dorsum of foot, posterior to fourth metatarsophalangeal joint, lateral side of tendon of extensor muscle of little toe
Posture: Supine
Angle: Oblique puncture
Direction: Toward sole
Depth: 8-10 mm
Indications: Dysmenorrhea, stomachalgia, suppression of lactation, deafness, mastitis

Point: Diwuhui
Meridian: GB 42
Location: On lateral side of dorsum of foot, posterior to fourth metatarsophalangeal joint, between fourth and fifth metatarsal bones, medial border of tendon of extensor muscle of little toe
Posture: Supine
Angle: Perpendicular puncture

Direction: Toward sole
Depth: 8-10 mm
Indications: Cholelithiasis, mastitis, conjunctivitis

Point: Xiaxi
Meridian: GB 43
Location: On lateral side of dorsum of foot, between fourth and fifth toes, proximal to margin of web
Posture: Supine
Angle: Perpendicular puncture
Direction: Toward sole
Depth: 5-10 mm

Indications: Dizziness, tinnitus, pain in chest and hypochondrium

Point: Zhuqiaoyin
Meridian: GB 44
Location: On lateral side of fourth toe, 0.1 *cun* proximal to corner of nail
Posture: Supine
Angle: Oblique puncture
Direction: Toward root of toe
Depth: 5 mm
Indications: Eye disorders, hypertension, insomnia, dreaminess, deafness

Appendix 3
Precautions in acupuncture treatment

1. The Lung Meridian of Head-Taiyin

When selecting Zhongfu (LU 1) and Yunmen (LU 2), these points should not be punctured deeply to avoid injuring the lung and resulting in pneumothorax. Shaoshang (LU 11) could be pricked with the three-edged needle to cause bleeding. It is inadvisable to apply direct moxibustion to the following points: Chize (LU 5), Jingqu (LU 8) and Taiyuan (LU 9).

2. The Large Intestine Meridian of Hand-Yangming

When the insertion is from Hegu (LI 4) to Laogong (PC 8), the needle should be toward the little finger. Puncture slowly to avoid internal hemorrhage by injuring an artery. Jugu (LI 16) should not be punctured deeply to avoid pneumothorax. Futu (LI 18) and Tianding (LI 17) should be punctured slowly to avoid injuring the carotid.

3. The Stomach Meridian of Foot-Yangming

Because there are many blood vessels in the face, it is important to puncture slowly the following points: Chengqi (ST 1), Sibai (ST 2), Juliao (ST 3), Dicang (ST 4), Daying (ST 5) and Jiache (ST 6), to avoid bleeding. There are also great vessels under Renying (ST 9), Shuitu (ST 10) and Qishe (ST 11) in the neck region, and these should not be punctured deeply. The thoracic cavity, heart and lung lie under Qihu (ST 13), Kufang (ST 14) and Wuyi (ST 15) in the chest; shallow insertion is advisable on these points. Also, it is advisable to puncture slowly, to lift and thrust the needle in frequently when puncturing points at the abdomen such as: Burong (ST 19), Chengman (ST 20), Liangmen (ST 21), Guanmen (ST 22), Taiyi (ST 23), Tianshu (ST 25), Wailing (ST 26), Daju (ST 27), Shuidao (ST 28), Guilai (ST 29), Qichong (ST 30). This will avoid injuring the internal organs. It is inadvisable to apply direct moxibustion to the face and joints, which may cause local scars and dysfunction.

4. The Spleen Meridian of Foot-Taiyin

To avoid injuring the heart and lungs, deep insertion of the needle is not advisable when puncturing at points in the chest: Dabao (SP 21), Zhourong (SP 20), Xiongxiang (SP 19), Tianxi (SP 18), Shidou (SP 17). When puncturing these points in the abdomen—Fujie (SP 14), Daheng (SP 15), Fubai (SP 16) and Fushe (SP 13)—it is advisable to lift and thrust the needle in frequently because of the stomach and intestine under these points.

5. The Heart Meridian of Hand-Shaoyin

On puncturing Jiquan (HT 1), the upper arm should be abducted to avoid puncturing the axillary artery. To avoid injuring the brachial artery, slow insertion is needed when puncturing at Qinling (HT 2). It is not advisable to apply direct moxibustion to the following points: Shaohai (HT 3), Yinxi (HT 6), Shenmen (HT 7) and Shaofu (HT 8).

6. The Small Intestine Meridian of Hand-Taiyang

When puncturing Jianzhen (SI 9) and Naoshu (SI 10), it is not advisable to insert deeply towards the chest. The direction of puncturing Bingfeng (SI 12) and Quyuan (SI 13) should be toward the superior of the supraclavicular fossa. To avoid impairing the lung, deep insertion is not advisable when puncturing Jianwaishu (SI 14) and Jianzhongshu (SI 15). Direct moxibustion is inadvisable when puncturing the following points: Qiangu (SI 2), Houxi (SI 3), Wangu (SI 4), Yanggu (SI 5), Quanliao (SI 18) and Tinggong (SI 19).

7. The Bladder Meridian of Foot-Taiyang

When puncturing Jingming (BL 1), it is advisable to insert the needle gently and to twirl it gently without lifting or thrusting; this can avoid impairing the ophthalmic artery and vein. To avoid injuring the internal organs, deep insertion is not advisable when puncturing the following points on the first lateral line at the back: Dashu (BL 11), Fengmen (BL 12), Feishu (BL 13), Xinshu (BL 15), Dushu (BL 16), Geshu (BL 17), Ganshu (BL 18), Danshu (BL 19), Pishu (BL 20), Weishu (BL 21), Sanjiaoshu (BL 22), Shenshu (BL 23), Qihaishu (BL 24), Dachangshu (BL 25), as well as these points on the second lateral line at the back: Fufen (BL 41), Pohu (BL 42), Gaohuang (BL 43), Shentang (BL 44), Yixi (BL 45), Geguan (BL 46), Hunmen (BL 47), Yanggang (BL 48), Yishe (BL 49), Weicang (BL 50), Huangmen (BL 51), and Zhishi (BL 52).

8. The Kidney Meridian of Foot-Shaoyin

To avoid injuring the internal organs, deep insertion is inadvisable when puncturing the following points on the chest: Shufu (KI 27), Yuzhong (KI 26), Shencang (KI 25), Lingxu (KI 24), Shenfeng (KI 23); and in the abdomen: Youmen (KI 21), Futonggu (KI 20), Yindu (KI 19), Shiguan (KI 18), Shangqu (KI 17), Huangshu (KI 16), Zhongzhu (KI 15), Siman (KI 14), Qixue (KI 13), Dahe (KI 12), and Henggu (KI 11).

9. The Pericardium Meridian of Hand-Jueyin

It is advisable to avoid injuring the median nerve when puncturing Neiguan (PC 6) and Jianshi (PC 5).

10. The Sanjiao Meridian of Hand-Shaoyang

It is inadvisable to puncture Tianyou (SJ 16) and Yifeng (SJ 17) too deeply and strongly. To avoid impairing the anterior auricular arteries, the patient's mouth should be open when Ermen (SJ 21) is punctured.

11. The Gallbladder Meridian of Foot-Shaoyang

It is advisable to avoid impairing the vertebral artery and the spinal cord when puncturing Riyue (GB 24), Yuanye (GB 22), and Zhejin (GB 23). Direct moxibustion should not be applied to points on the face and head.

12. The Liver Meridian of Foot-Jueyin

To avoid injuring the liver, deep insertion is not advisable when puncturing Qimen (LR 14) and Zhangmen (LR 13).

13. The Du Meridian

To avoid injuring the rectum, it is advisable to puncture with an angle of approximately 45 degrees with the skin surface upward along the anterior border of the coccyx. It is advisable to puncture perpendicularly these points between the spinous process: Dazhui (DU 14) and Taodao (DU 13) on the neck region, and Jizhong (DU 6), Xuanshu (DU 5), Mingmen (DU 4) and Yaoyangguan (DU 3) on the lumbus. It is advisable to puncture obliquely upwards 0.5-1 *cun* the following points on the chest: Shenzhu (DU 12), Shendao (DU 11), Lingtai (DU 10), Zhiyang (DU 9), Jinsuo (DU 8), and Zhongshu (DU 7). To avoid injuring the medullary bulb, when puncturing Yamen (DU 15) and Fengfu (DU 16) it is advisable to puncture slowly and obliquely towards the lower jaw; deep and upward puncturing is controindicated.

14. The Ren Meridian

To avoid injuring the internal organs, deep insertion is inadvisable when puncturing the points in the chest and abdomen. Shenque (RN 8) should not be punctured; instead, moxibustion is applicable. Caution should be followed in applying the following points to pregnant women: Yinjiao (RN 7), Qihai (RN 6), Shimen (RN 5) and Guanyuan (RN 4). To avoid injuring the liver, deep insertion is inadvisable when puncturing Juque (RN 14) and Jiuwei (RN 15). Before Zhongji (RN 3) or Guanyuan (RN 4) are punctured, the patient should urinate to avoid injury to the bladder or the womb by deep insertion, especially pregnant women. It is advisable to puncture horizontally upward or downward. Danzhong (RN 17) is punctured horizontally toward the base of the breast. Electroacupuncture apparatus should not be used. To avoid injuring the subclavian artery and the apex of the lung, when puncturing Tiantu (RN 22) it is advisable to puncture between the trachea and the sternum; deep insertion and/or slanted needle are inadvisable.

Appendix 4
The selected points in acupuncture treatment of common diseases

1. Common cold

Prescription: Fengchi, Hegu, Lieque, Dazhui.
Point Modification—nasal obstruction: add Yingxiang, Shangxing.
Headache: add Taiyang, Baihui.
Sore throat: add spot pricking Shaoshang, Yuji.
High fever: add Quchi, Waiguan.

2. Cough

Prescription:
1) Exopathogenic cough: Feishu, Lieque, Hegu, Fengchi, Dazhui.
Point Modification—Laryngalgia: add Shaoshang, Chize.
High fever: add Dazhui, Waiguan.
2) Endopathogenic cough: (a) phlegm-dampness: Feishu, Chize, Zhangmen, Taibai, Fenglong, Zusanli. (b) cough due to liver-fire: Feishu, Chize, Yanglingquan, Taichong.
Point Modification-forehead pain: add Yangbai, Yintang, Cuanzhu.

3. Headache

Prescription: Baihui, Fengchi, Taiyang, Hegu, Fengmen, Xiangu, Shangxing, Touwei.
Migraine: add penetration needling from Taiyang to Shuaigu, Sidu, Waiguan, Zulinqi, Xiaxi. Occipital headache: add Houxi, Jingmen, Shugu, Fengfu, Houding, Tianzhu, Kunlun.
Pain in the vertex: add Neiguan, Taichong, Yongquan, Tongtian, Xingjian. Exopathic wind: add Hegu, Lieque, Feishu. Hyperactivity of the liver-*yang*: add Sanyinjiao, Taichong, Linqi, Fengchi, Lieque, Xuanlu, Xiaxi, Xingjian. Stagnation of phlegm-dampness in middle Jiao: add Zhongwan, Fenglong, Zusanli. Deficiency of *Qi*: add Qihai, Shangxing, Ganshu.

4. Bronchitis

Prescription: Tiantu, Dingchuan, Lieque, Feishu.

Point Modification—exopathogenic fever: add Hegu. Choking sensation in chest: add Neiguan. Abundant expectoration: add Fenglong, Zusanli.
(Note: Dingchuan is 0.5 *cun* lateral to Dazhui.)

5. Asthma

Prescription: Dingchuan, Feishu, Tiantu, Danzhong, Taiyuan, Guanyuan.
Point Modification—deficiency syndrome of the lung: add Zhongfu, Pianli. Deficiency of the kidney: add Zhongfu, Taixi.
Exopathogen: add Hegu, Fenglong. Stagnation of phlegm in the lung: add Zusanli, Zhongwan, Fenglong.

6. Insomnia

Prescription: Shenmen, Sanyinjiao.
Point Modification—deficiency of heart and spleen: Xinshu, Jueyinshu, Pishu, Tongli, Shenmen. Timidity due to deficiency of heart and gall bladder: Xinshu, Danshu, Daling, Xuehai.
Disharmony between the heart and kidney: Xinshu, Shenshu, Taixi.
Abnormal rise of the liver-*Yang*: Ganshu, Jianshi, Taichong, Dadun. Incoordination between spleen and stomach: Weishu, Zusanli, Gongsun, Shenmen.

7. Stomachalgia (Gastritis, Gastric Ulcer, Gastroneurosis)

Prescription: Zhongwan, Zusanli, Hegu, Neiguan, Taichong, Guanyuan.
Point Modification—the hyperactive liver-*Qi* attacking the stomach: add Qimen, Yanglingquan. Insufficiency of the spleen-*Yang*: add Pishu, Weishu, Zhangmen.

8. Gastroptosis

Prescription: Zusanli, Weishangxue, the penetration needling from Zhongwan to Xiawan.
Note: Weishangxue is 2 *cun* above the umbilicus, 4 *cun* lateral to the midline of the abdomen.

9. Abdominalgia

Prescription: Hegu, Zusanli, Sanyinjiao.
Point Modification—the pain in region above umbilicus: add Zhongwan, Liangmen, Taichong. Pain in region below umbilicus: add Guanyuan, Zhongji, Xiawan. Periumbilical pain: add Tianshu, Qihai, Fenglong. Pain of the lateral aspect of abdomen: add Yanglingquan. Chronic pain: add Pishu, Weishu, Tianshu.
Accumulation of cold in the interior: Zhongwan, Shenque, Guanyuan, Zusanli, Gongsun. Deficiency of spleen-*Yang*: Pishu, Weishu, Zhongwan, Qihai, Zhangmen, Zusanli. Retention of food: Zhongwan, Tianshu, Zusanli, Qihai, Neiting.

10. Diarrhea

Prescription: Zhongwan, Tianshu, Zusanli, Guanyuan.
Point Modification—acute diarrhea: add Shangjuxu, Yinlingquan.
Chronic diarrhea: add Pishu, Zhangmen. Deficiency of the kidney: add Mingmen, Taixi, Shenshu, Feiyang.

11. Acute Enteritis

Prescription: Tianshu, Zusanli, Shangjuxu, Yinlingquan.
Point Modification—abdominalgia: add Hegu, Sanyinjiao. Nausea and vomiting: add Neiguan. Fever: add Quchi. Tenesmus: add Guanyuan.

12. Dysentery

Prescription: Zhongwan, Zusanli, Dachangshu.
Point-Modification—dysentery of cold nature: add Pishu, Weishu, Zhongwan (with moxibustion), Zusanli (with moxibustion), Hegu, Lieque. Dysentery of hot nature: add Neiting, Tianshu, Wenliu.

13. Vomiting (gastritis, hepatitis, cardiospasm, pylorospasm, pylorochesis, pancreatitis, cholecystitis)

Prescription: Zhongwan, Weishu, Zusanli, Neiguan.
Point-Modification—vomiting of hot nature: add Hegu, Jinjin, Yuye, Shangwan, Neiting. Vomiting of cold nature: add Shangwan, Taibai, Fenglong. Due to phlegm retention: add Danzhong, Fenglong. Due to dyspepsia: add Xiawan, Xuanji, Chongyang. Due to liver-*Qi*: add Yanglingquan, Taichong, Ganshu. Due to deficiency of *Qi* in middle-Jiao: add Pishu, Zhangmen.

14. Diabetes

Prescription: Feishu, Hegu, Zusanli, Taiyuan.
Point-Modification—diabetes involving the upper-Jiao: add Chize, Yuji, Lianquan, Pianli. Diabetes involving the middle-Jiao: add Pishu, Shangwan, Neiting, Weishu, Chongyang. Diabetes involving the lower-Jiao: add Sanjiaoshu, Guanyuan, Sanyinjiao, Shenshu, Taixi.

15. Dizziness

Prescription: Fengchi, Taichong, Hegu, Ganshu, Shenshu, Sanyinjiao.
Point-Modification—due to deficiency of *Qi* and blood: add Qihai, Zusanli, Pishu, Baihui, Gongsun. Due to phlegm-dampness obstruction in the middle-Jiao: add Zhongwan, Fenglong, Neiguan, Jiexi, Touwei, Fengchi, Shangxing, Taiyang, Hegu. Due to hyperactivity of liver-*Yang*: add Xingjian, Xiaxi.

16. Palpitation

Prescription: 1) Shenmen, Neiguan, Sanyinjiao; 2) Xinshu, Zusanli. The points of both groups could be used alternately.
Point-Modification—fast heart rate: add Jianshi. Slow heart rate: add Suliao. Choking sensation in chest: add Danzhong. Phlegm-dampness: add Fenglong.

17. Heliosis

Prescription: 1) Quchi, Neiguan, Renzhong, Dazhui. 2) Weizhong, Shixuan, Renzhong, Quze.
Point-Modification—myospasm: add Yanglingquan.

18. Phrenospasm

Prescription: 1) Neiguan, Tiantu, Fenglong. 2) Geshu, Zusanli, Chongyang. 3) Danzhong, Taichong, Zhongwan, Gongsun. The points of three groups could be used alternately.

19. Hepatitis

Prescription: 1) Yanggang, Zhiyang, Yinlingquan. 2) Ganshu, Danshu, Pishu, Yanglingquan. 3) Zusanli, Taichong, Sanyinjiao.
Point-Modification—nausea and vomiting: add Neiguan. Abdominal distension: add Tianshu, Qihai. Fever: add Dazhui, Quchi. Hypochodriac pain: add Zhigou.

20. Jaundice

Prescription: Danshu, Zusanli, Taichong, Sanyinjiao.
Point-Modification—*yang*-type jaundice: add Yanglingquan, Yinlingquan, Neiting. Chest tightness and nausea: add Neiguan, Gongsun. Abdominal distension and constipation: add Dachangshu, Tianshu. *Yin*-type jaundice: add Zhiyang, Pishu, Danshu, Zhongwan.
General lassitude and aversion to cold: add Mingmen, Qihai. Loose stool: add Tianshu, Guanyuan.

21. Hydrops

Prescription: Shuifen, Qihai, Sanjiaoshu, Zusanli.
Point-Modification—*yang*-type: add Feishu, Hegu, Renzhong, Fengchi, Fengmen, Zhongfu. *Yin*-type: add Pishu, Shenshu, Yinlingquan, Zhangmen, Taixi, Feiyang.

22. Abdominal Distension

Prescription: Zhongwan, Qihai, Sanyinjiao.

Point-Modification—stagnation of the liver-*Qi*: add Taichong, Qimen. Blood stasis in interior: add Xiawan, Xuehai, Zhongdu.
Indigestion and stagnation of phlegm: add Shangwan, Liangmen, Gongsun.

23. Constipation

Prescription: Dachangshu, Tianshu, Zhigou, Shangjuxu.
Point-Modification—heat type: add Hegu, Quchi. *Qi* stagnation type: add Zhongwan, Xingjian. Deficiency of *Qi* and blood: add Pishu, Weishu, Qihai, Zusanli. Cold type: add Shenque (with moxibustion), Qihai, Weishu, Chongyang.

24. Rheumatic Heart Disease

Prescription: Neiguan, Jianshi, Ximen, Xinshu, Shaofu.
Point-Modification—atrial fibrillation: add Chize, Quze, Daling. Ascites: add penetration needling from Zhongji to Qugu and Shuiquan, penetration needling from Yinlingquan to Yanglingquan. Inappetence, nausea, vomiting: add Zhongwan, Zusanli.

25. Pulmonary Tuberculosis

Prescription: Chize, Feishu, Gaohuang, Zusanli.
Point-Modification—inappetence: add Pishu, Zhongwan. Tidal fever: add Dazhui, Taixi. Night sweats: add Yinxi, Fuliu. Hemoptysis: add Yuji, Geshu, Kongzui, Taixi. Spermatorrhea: add Zhishi, Guanyuan, Sanyinjiao. Amenorrhea: add Xuehai, Pishu.

26. Haematemesis

Prescription: Weishu, Neiguan, Hegu, Daling, Shenmen, Yuji.
Point-Modification—stomach-neat: add Neiting, Liangqiu. Insufficiency of the spleen: add Zusanli, Yinbai, Fenglong, Diji. Stagnation of the liver-*Qi*: add Ganshu, Taichong.

27. Hypertension

Prescription: 1) Quchi, Zusanli, Taiyang. 2) Hegu, Taichong, Fengchi.
Point-Modification—tinnitus: add Waiguan, Yifeng. Insomnia: add Shenmen, Sanyinjiao. Palpitation: add Neiguan. Phlegm-dampness: add Zhongwan, Fenglong.

28. Meniere's Syndrome

Prescription: 1) Fengchi, Neiguan, Yanglingquan. 2) Yifeng, Sanyinjiao, Zusanli. The points of both groups could be used alternately.

29. Shock

Prescription: Renzhong, Zhongchong, Zusanli, Neiguan, Yongquan, Suliao.

30. Apoplexy

Prescription: excess syndrome of apoplexy: Shuigou, 12 Jing-well points, Taichong, Fenglong, Baihui, Yongquan, Laogong. (Note: The 12 Jiang-well points are *Yin* Meridian's Shaoshang, Yongquan, Dadun, Shaochong, Yinbai, Zhongchong; and *Yang* Meridian's Shangyang, Zhiyin, Zuqiaoyin, Shaoze, Lidui, Guanchong.)
Prostration syndrome: Guanyuan, Shenque, Zusanli, Neiguan. Hemiparalysis: upper limb: Jianyu, Quchi, Shousanli, Waiguan, Hegu. Lower limb: Huantiao, Yanglingquan, Zusanli, Jiexi, Kunlun.
Point-Modification—slurred speech: add lianquan, Tongli, Yamen. Deviation of the mouth: Dicang, Jiache, Hegu, Neiting, Taichong. Disapperance of nasolabial sulcus: add Yingxiang, Heliao. Deviation of nasolabial sulcus: add Shuigou. Deviation of mentolabial sulcus: add Chengjiang. Ophthalmoplegia: Sibai, Cuanzhu, Shenmai, Zhaohai. Stiffness of musculi faciales: add Sibai, Juliao. Long course of disease: add Dazhui, Jianwaishu, Yaoyangguan, Baihuanshu. Spasm of cubitus: add Quze. Spasm of wrist: add Daling. Spasm of knee: add Ququan. Spasm of ankle: add Taixi.

31. Hematochezia

Prescription: Guanyuan, Zusanli, Fenglong, Neiting, Tianshu, Pishu, Sanyinjiao.
Point-Modification—deficiency syndrome: Guanyuan (with Moxibustion), Zusanli (with Moxibustion), Taibai, Diji. Excess syndrome: add Shangjuxu, Dachangshu, Hegu, Lieque, Wenliu.

32. Hematuria

Prescription: Sanyinjiao, Qihai, Zhongji, Mingmen, Guanyuan.
Point-Modification—the moving downwards of the liver-fire: add Ganshu, Taichong, Pangguangshu. Damp-heat in the urinary bladder: add Yinlingquan, Jinmen. Hypofunction of the spleen and kidney: Guanyuan (with Moxibustion), Zusanli (with Moxibustion), Taibai, Fenglong.

33. Proctoptosis

Prescription: Changqiang, Weishu, Zusanli, Dachangshu, Tianshu, Baihui.
Point-Modification—heat of excess type in the large intestine: add Dazhui, Neiting, Hegu, Lieque, Chengshan. Collapse of the spleen-*Qi*: add Pishu, Zhangmen, Taibai, Fenglong, Qihai.

34. Malaria

Prescription: 1) Dazhui, Jianshi, Zusanli. 2) Taodao, Houxi, Quchi. The points of both groups could be used alternately.

35. Hernia

Prescription: 1) Qihai, Guanyuan, Sanyinjiao. 2) Zhongdu, Yanglingquan, Taichong. The points of both groups could be used alternately.

36. Palpitation

Prescription: Ximen, Shenmen, Xinshu, Juque.
Point-Modification—deficiency of heart blood: Geshu, Pishu, Zusanli, Zhizheng. Internal disturbance due to phlegm-fire: Chize, Neiguan, Fenglong, Zusanli, Taibai. Accumulation of excessive fluid in the body: Pishu, Weishu, Sanjiaoshu, Taixi, Feiyang.

37. Neurasthenia

Prescription: 1) Shenmen, Neiguan, Sanyinjiao. 2) Anmian, Zusanli. (Note: Anmian is at the midpoint of the line joining Yifeng and Fengchi.)
Point-Modification—headache and dizziness: add Fengchi, Baihui, Taiyang. Hypomnesis and tiredness: add Ganshu, Danshu, Pishu, Shenshu, Sanyinjiao.

38. Hysteria

Prescription: Renzhong, Yamen, Neiguan, Sanyinjiao, Hegu, Taichong.
Point-Modification—hypnopompic state: add Yongquan, Renzhong.
Mental confusion: add Yamen, Renzhong, Neiguan. Convulsion of the extremities: add Houxi, Sanyinjiao, Renzhong. Paralysis of limb: add Quchi, Yanglingquan. Obstruction of throat: add Tiantu, Lianquan. Aphasia: add Yamen, Lianquan, Tongli.

39. Schizophrenia

Prescription: 1) Renzhong, Hegu, Taichong, Jianshi, Daling, Shenmen. 2) Taiyang, Neiguan, Sanyinjiao, Fenglong, Fengfu, Jiuwei. 3) Yamen, Dazhui, Taodao, Shenzhu, Ganshu, Xinshu. The points of three groups could be used alternately.

40. Epilepsy

Prescription: 1) Renzhong, Shaoshang, Houxi, Shenmai, Dazhui, Xinshu. 2) Hegu, Taichong, Juque, Baihui, Yongquan. The above groups could be used in the stage of attack. 3) Yamen, Zhongwan, Neiguan, Danzhong. 4) Xinshu, Ganshu, Pishu, Fenglong, Shenmen. 5) Jiuwei, Yaoqi, Fengfu, Jianshi. (Yaoqi is at 2 *cun* above the tip of the coccyx.) The last 3 groups could be used in the normal stage.

41. Trigeminal Neuralgia

Prescription: the first branch: Cuanzhu, the penetration needling from Taiyang to Shuaigu, Yangbai, Yuyao, Sanjian. (Note: Yuyao is midway between eyebrows.) The second branch: Sibai, Taiyang, Juliao, Quanliao. The thrid branch: Xiaquan, Chengjiang, Jiache. Alternate points: 1) Hegu, Neiting, Yangfu. 2) Waiguan, Zulinqi, Fengchi, Taichong.

42. Facial Paralysis

Prescription: Yangbai, Cuanzhu, Sibai, Dicang, Jiache, Xiaguan, Quanliao, Hegu, Taichong, Zusanli, Fengchi.
Point-Modification—disapperance of nasolabial sulcus: add Yingxiang, Heliao. Ophthalmoplegia: Yangbai, Shenmai, Zhaohai. Disapperance of philtrum: add Renzhong. Deviation of mentolabial sulcus: add Chengjiang, Shuigou. Mastodealgia: add Yifeng, Fengchi. Stiffness of musculi faciales: add Juliao.

43. Facial Spasm

Prescription: Sibai, Dicang, Quanliao, Hegu, Taichong.

44. Hypochondriac pain

Prescription: 1) Zhigou, Yanglingquan, Qimen. 2) Neiguan, Taichong, Zusanli, Ganshu. The two groups could be used alternately.

45. Sciatica

Prescription: Huantiao, Zhibian, Yingmen, Yanglingquan. Alternate points: Shangliao, Weizhong, Chengshan, Houxi, Zhongzhu.

46. Paraplegia

Prescription: 1) Huatuojiaji. 2) Ciliao, Zhibian, Yinlian, Weizhong, Zusanli, Sanyinjiao.

47. Mononeuritis Multiplex

Prescription: Quchi, Waiguan, Hegu, Zusanli, Juegu, Sanyinjiao.

48. Brachial Plexus Neuralgia

Prescription: Tianzong, Jianyu, Jianliao, Quchi, Waiguan, Hegu, Houxi, Jianzhen, Zhizheng.

49. Peripheral Nerve Injury

Prescription: Radial Nerve: Jianyu, Binao, Quchi, Shousanli, Waiguan, Lieque, Hegu. Ulnar nerve: Jianzhen, Shaohai, Zhizheng, Houxi, Shenmen, Yanggu, Tongli, Zhongzhu, Shaoze, Guanchong. Median nerve: Chize, Quze, Ximen, Neiguan, Hegu, Kongzui. Common peroneal nerve: Yanglingquan, Zusanli, Juegu, Jiexi, Qiuxu.

50. Rheumatism

Prescription: nigratory arthralgia (wandering pain, without fixed place): Geshu, Xuehai. Arthralgia aggravated by cold (arthrodynia, in fixed place): Shenshu, Guanyuan. Damp arthralgia (aching pain, in fixed place): Zusanli, Shangqiu. Arthralgia of heat type: Dazhui, Quchi. Shoulder: Jianyu, Jianliao, Naoshu. Elbow: Quchi, Hegu, Tianjing, Waiguan, Chize. Wrist: Yangchi, Waiguan, Yangxi, Wangu. Spine: Shuigou, Shenzhu, Yaoyangguan, Huatuojiaji. Hip: Huantiao, Juliao, Xuanzhong. Thigh: Zhibian, Chengfu, Fengshi, Yanglingquan. Knee: Dubi, Liangqiu, Yanglingquan, Xiyangguan. Ankle: Shenmai, Zhaohai, Kunlun, Qiuxu.

51. Periarthritis of Shoulder

Prescription: Jianyu, Jianliao, Tiaokou, Yanglingquan.
Point-Modification—upper arm pain: add Binao, Quchi. Scapulalgia: add Quyuan, Tianzong.

52. Lumbago

Prescription: 1) Ashi, Huatuojiaji, Weizhong. 2) Yanglao, Renzhong. 3) Shenshu, Mingmen, Yaoyangguan, Taixi, Feiyang. 4) Zhishi, Weizhong, Fengchi, Zhongdu, Shuiquan. The above groups could be used alternately.
Point-Modification—pain of spine: add Shenzhu, Jizhong, Shenshu, Weizhong, Kunlun.

53. Myasthenia (Myoatrophy)

Prescription: upper limb: Jianyu, Quchi, Hegu, Yangxi, Dazhui, Jianjing, Jianliao, Bingfeng, Lieque. Lower limb: Biguan, Liangqiu, Zusanli, Jiexi, Neiting, Huantiao, Sanyinjiao. Select 3-5 points every time: treat every second day.
Point-Modification—for lung heat: add Chize, Feishu, Dazhui. Damp heat: add Yinlingquan, Pishu. Deficiency of liver-*Yin* and kidney-*Yin*: Ganshu, Shenshu, Xuanzhong, Yanglingquan.

54. Enuresis

Prescription: 1) Guanyuan, Sanyinjiao, Zusanli, Taixi, Feiyang, Zhongji. 2) Shenshu, Pangguangshu, Ciliao, Jinggu, Dazhong.

55. Anuresis

Prescription: 1) Guanyuan, Zhongji, Sanyinjiao, Sanjiaoshu, Qihai. 2) Pangguang-shu, Ciliao, Yinlingquan, Dazhong, Jinggu.

56. Spermatorrhea

Prescription: 1) Guanyuan, Zusanli, Taixi, Jingmen. 2) Shenshu, Zhishi, Sanyin-jiao, Shenmen.

57. Impotence

Prescription: Qihai, Guanyuan (with moxibustion), Mingmen (with Moxibustion), Sanyinjiao, Taixi, Fengyang.

58. Urinary System Infection

Prescription: 1) Zhongji, Ququan. 2) Ciliao, Sanyinjiao.
Point-Modification—urodynia: add Xingjian. Lumbago: add Shenshu. Fever: add Quchi.

59. Nephritis

Prescription: 1) Shenshu, Sanyinjiao. 2) Guanyuan, Yinlingquan, Zusanli. 3) Shuifen, Pishu, Fuliu, Lieque. The points of three groups could be used alternately.

60. Acute Appendicitis

Prescription: Tianshu, Lanwei, Zhongwan, Quchi, Zusanli, Shangjuxu. (Lanwei is 2 *cun* below Zusanli.)
Point-Modification—fever: add Quchi, Neiting.

61. Disorders of Biliary Tract

Prescription: 1) Dannang, Neiguan. (Dannang is 1 *cun* below Yanglingquan.) 2) Zusanli, the penetration needling from Yingxiang to Sibai, Yanglingquan. 3) Ganshu or Huatuojiaji (0.5 *cun* lateral to inferior to the spinous process of the first to fifth thoracic vertebrae).

62. Gastric and Duodenal Ulcer

Prescription: Zhongwan, Tianshu, Zusanli, Neiguan.

63. Parotitis

Prescription: Jiache, Xiaguan, Hegu, Jiaosun.

64. Mastitis

Prescription: Jianjing, Rugen, Zusanli, Zulingqi, Danzhong, Shaoze, Chongyang, Neiting, Gongsun.
Point-Modification—fever: add Hegu, Quchi.

65. Arthritis

Prescription: 1) Mandibular joint: Xiaguan, Hegu. 2) Spondylarthritis: Huatuojia-ji, Yinmen, Weizhong, Dazhui. 3) Omarthritis: Jianyu, Jianliao. 4) Elbow: Quchi, Shaohai, Tianjing. 5) The wrist joint, metacarpophalangeal articulation: Yangchi, Daling, Zhongquan (at the center of wrist, in the depression of the radial side of the tendon of the common extensor muscle of fingers.) 6) Lumbosacral joint: Yaoyangguan, Huatuojiaji. 7) Sacro-ilitis: Dachangshu, Xiaochangshu. 8) Coxitis: Huantiao, Juliao. 9) Gonitis: Xiyan, Liangqiu, Yanglingquan. (Note: Xiyan is in the depression on the lateral side of apex patellae.) 10) Ankle joint: Jiexi, Qiuxu, Taixi.
Point-Modification—fever in the acute stage: add Dazhui, Quchi. Tranquilizing the mind and dispelling wind and dampness: add Neiguan, Xuehai, Sanyinjiao. Analgesia: add Hegu, Taichong.

66. Erysipelas

Prescription: Dazhui, Quchi, Weizhong, Xuehai.

67. Furuncle

Prescription: Lingtai, Shenshu, Weizhong, Hegu.
Point-Modification—invagination: add Laogong, Shenmen.

68. Acute Lymphangitis

Prescription: Quze, Weizhong, Shixuan, Ashi. (Note: Shixuan is at the tip of finger, 0.1 *cun* from nail.)

69. Tetanus

Prescription: Yamen, Dazhui, Jinsuo, Fengchi.
Point-Modification—gnathospasmus: Xiaguan, Jiache, Hegu. Opisthotonus: Renzhong, Yaoyangguan, Houxi, Shenmai, Changqiang, Yongquan, Shuigou, Chengshan, Kunlun. Convulsion of the extremities: Quchi, Yanglingquan, Taichong, Hegu, Houxi, Waiguan.

70. Tuberculosis of Lymph Node

Prescription: Ganshu, Geshu, Ashi.
Point-Modification—cervical lymph node: add penetration needling from Binao to Quchi, Shousanli. Nape lymph node: add Yifeng, Tianjing, Zhigou, Zulingqi. Subzxilla lymph node: add Jianjing, Shaohai, Fuyang.

71. Piles

Prescription: Changqing, Chengshan, Yinjiao, Erbai (4 *cun* directly above the centre of the carpal crease, and both lateral sides of the tendon of the radial fiexor muscle of wrist).
Point-Modification—constipation: add Dachangshu, Zhigou.

72. Urticaria

Prescription: 1) Quchi, Xuehai, Sanyinjiao. 2) Geshu, Zusanli.

73. Neurodermatitis

Prescription: 1) Quchi, Xuehai, Ashi. 2) Huatuojiaji.

74. Stiff Neck

Prescription: 1) Fengchi, Houxi, Ashi. 2) Juegu, Lochen (in the dorsum of hand between the second and third metacarpal bone, 0.5 *cun* posterior to metacarpophalangeal articulation).

75. Omalgia

Prescription: penetration needling from Tiaokou to Chengshan, Jugu, Bingfeng, Quchi, Waiguan, Ashi.
Point-Modification—Scapulohumeral periarthritis: add Tianzong, Naoshu. Tendinitis of supraspinatus muscle: add Jianyu, Jugu. Subacromial bursitis: add Jianyu, Jianliao. Tenovaginitis of brachial biceps: add Jianyu, Quchi.

76. Elbow Pain

Prescription: 1) Tender spot, Quchi, Zhouliao, Yanglingquan, Tianjing. 2) Choosing points of right side to treat disorder of the left, and vice versa. Wrist joint: Wangu, Yangxi, Yangchi.

77. Disorders of Tendon Sheath of Wrist

Prescription: Ahshi.
Point-Modification—tenosynovitis stenosans: add Yangxi, Lieque. Carpal tunnel

syndrome: Daling, Neiguan, Baxie (on the dorsum posterior border of the webs between the fingers of the hands).

78. Tenvaginitis of Flexor Digitorum

Prescription: Ahshi.
Point-Modification—pain in thumb: add Lieque. Pain in index and middle fingers: add Daling. Pain in ring and little fingers: add Shenmen.

79. Soft Tissue Injury of Knee Region

Prescription: Tender spot, Weizhong, penetrating needling from Xiyangguan to Ququan, Xiyang (a pair of points at the depression on both medial and lateral sides to apex of patella).

80. Soft Tissue Injury of Ankle Region

Prescription: 1) Tender spot, Juegu. 2) Zhongquan, Yanggu.

81. Painful Heels

Prescription: 1) Tender spot, Taixi. 2) Daling.

82. Thyropathy

Prescription: Ahshi, Hegu, Naohui.
Point-Modification—hoarseness: add Tiantu. Flaring heart-fire and liver fire: add Taichong, Neiguan, Sanyinjiao.

83. Menoxenia

Prescription: 1) Guanyuan, Sanyinjiao, Zusanli, Taixi, Fengyang. 2) Qihai, Xuehai, Yinlingquan, Xingjian. 3) Ganshu, Pishu, Ciliao, Zhangmen, Qimen. The three groups could be used alternately.

84. Amenorrhea

Prescription: 1) Blood depletion: Weishu, Zhongwan, Qihai, Shenshu (with moxibustion), Xuehai, Zusanli (with moxibustion), Sanyinjiao, Taibai, Fenglong. 2) Stagnation of blood: Zhongji, Qihai, Xuehai, Sanyinjiao, Taichong, Guangming.

85. Dysmenorrhea

Prescription: 1) Guanyuan, Sanyinjiao, Qihai, Xuehai. 2) Zhongji, Diji, Taichong. 3) Ciliao, Hegu.

86. Metrorrhagia

Prescription: Guanyuan, Sanyinjiao, Yinbai, Zusanli, Dadun.
Point-Modification—pathogenic heat: Qihai, Xuehai, Ganshu, Qimen. Deficiency of Qi: Guanyuan (with moxibustion), Zusanli (with moxibustion), Taibai, Fenglong. Blood stasis: Qihai, Zhongji, Geshu, Taichong, Guangming.

87. Leukorrhea

Prescription: 1) Qihai, Weidao, Sanyinjiao. 2) Ganshu, Pishu, Ciliao.
Point-Modification—damp-heat: add Xingjian, Yinlingquan. Cold-dampness: add Guanyuan, Zusanli.

88. Pelvic Information

Prescription: 1) Acute pelvic inflammation: Zhongji, Guilai, Sanyinjiao. 2) Chronic pelvic inflammation: Baliao, Shenshu, Zusanli.

89. Hysteroptosis

Prescription: 1) Weidao, Sanyinjiao, Guanyuan. 2) Qihai, Baihui, Zusanli.

90. Impotence

Prescription: Shenshu, Mingmen, Sanyinjiao, Guanyuan.

91. Morning Sickness (a group of symptoms including nausea, vomiting and inappetence, a commonly seen disorder appearing during early stages of pregnancy)

Prescription: Neiguan, Zusanli, Chengjiang, Taichong.

92. Abnormal Fetal Position

Prescription: Zhiyin.

93. Prolonged Labour

Prescription: Sanyinjiao, Taichong, Hegu, Zhiyin, Zusanli, Taibai, Fenglong.

94. Postpartum Syncope

Prescription: Shuigou, Baihui, Zhongchong, Zusanli, Taibai, Fenglong.

95. Placenta Praevia

Prescription: Qihai, Xuehai, Hegu, Sanyinjiao, Zusanli.

96. Hypogalactia

Prescription: Danzhong, Rugen, Shaoze, Zusanli.

97. Fever in Children

Prescription: 1) Exopathy: Dazhui, Fengmen, Fengchi, Hegu, Lieque. 2) Dyspepsia: Shangyang, Guanchong, Zusanli.

98. Chin Cough

Prescription: 1) Tiantu, Dingchuan (0.5 *cun* lateral to Dazhui). 2) Neiguan, Sifeng (on the palmar surface, at the mid-point of the transverse crease of the distal interphalangeal joints of the index, middle, ring and little fingers). 3) Dazhui, Shenzhu, Hegu, Fenglong.

99. Dyspepsia in Children

Prescription: 1) Sifeng (spot pricking with a three-edged needle). 2) Tianshu, Zusanli, Pishu, Weishu.
Point Modification—vomiting: add Neiguan. Abdominalgia: add Qihai. Abdominal Distension: add Pishu, Gongsun. Fever: add Dazhui, Sanyinjiao.

100. Infantile Convulsion

Prescription: Renzhong, Shixuan (on the tips of the ten tingers, about 0.1 *cun* distal to the nail).
Point Modification—fever: add Dazhui, Quchi. Lockjaw: add Jiache. Convulsion of extremities: add Houxi, Shemai, Yanglingquan. Opisthotonus: add Fengchi, Shenzhu, Taichong. Abundant expertoration: add Lieque, Fenglong. Coma: add Yongquan.

101. Poliomyelitis

Prescription: Jianyu, Binao, Quchi, Waiguan, Hegu, Huantiao, Zhibian, Yinmen, Fengshi, Zusanli, Yanglingquan, Juegu, Kunlun, Sanyinjiao, Pishu, Weishu, Ganshu, Shenshu. About 3-6 points in a diseased region could be punctured with strong stimulation every time.

102. Acute Conjunctivitis

Prescription: 1) Fengchi, Taiyang, Hegu, Jingming. 2) Erjian bleeding by spot

pricking.
Point Modification—pathogenic wind-heat: add Shaoshang, Shangxing. Excessive fire in the liver and the gallbladder: add Xiaxi.

103. Myopia

Prescription: 1) Penetrating needling from Chengqi to Jingming. 2) Yiming, Fengchi, Guangming, Hegu. Select 2 points every time. (Yiming is 1 *cun* posterior to Yifeng.)

104. Glaucoma

Prescription: Qiuhou (between the junction of the lateral 1/4 and the medial 3/4 of the infraorbitalmargin and eyeball), Jingming, Fengchi.
Point Modification—headache: add Taiyang. Ophthalmalgia: add Cuanzhu. Nausea and vomiting: add Neiguan. For reduction of intraocular pressure: add Xingjian, Sanyinjiao.

105. Disorders of Eyeground (Optic Atrophy, Central Retinitis, Pigmentary Degeneration of Retina)

Prescription: 1) Jingming, Qiuhou, Yiming. 2) Ganshu, Shenshu, Xingjian, Sanyinjiao, Fengchi.

106. Tonsillitis, Pharyngitis

Prescription: Tianrong, Hegu, Neiting, Shaoshang.
Point Modification—fever: add Dazhui, Qichi.

107. Nasosinusitis

Prescription: Yingxiang, Hegu, Lieque.
Point Modification—headache, dizziness: add Yintang, Fengchi, Cuanzhu.

108. Toothache

Prescription: 1) Hegu, Neiting. 2) Taiyang.
Point Modification—wind-fire: add Waiguan, Fengchi. Deficiency of the kidney: add Zhaohai, Xingjian. Upper toothache: add Xiaguan, Neiting, Quanliao. Lower toothache: add Jiache, Dicang.

109. Deafness

Prescription: Ermen, Tinggong, Tinghui, Yifeng, Zhongzhu, Waiguan.
Point Modification—excessive fire in the liver and the gallbladder: add Taichong, Qiuxu. Expathic wind: add Waiguan, Hegu. Deficiency of the kidney: add Shenshu,

Guanyuan.

110. Alalia

Prescription: Yamen, Lianquan, Tongli, Ermen, Tinggong, Tinghui, Fengfu, Wai-guan, Hegu, Zhongzhu. Select 3-5 points every time, alternately using above points. Retain the needle about 10-20 minutes, with treatment every second day.

111. Tinnitus

Prescription: Ermen, Yifeng, Zhongzhu, Tinggong, Tinghui.
Point Modification—dyssomnia by tinnitus: add Taixi. Dizziness: add Taichong.

112. Nasal Obstruction

Prescription: Fengchi, Hegu, Shangxing, Yingxiang, Taiyuan, Pianli.

113. Rhinorrhagia

Prescription: Wind-head: Fengmen, Shaoshang, Dazhui, Taiyuan, Pianli, Yingxiang. Stomach-fire: Hegu, Erjian, Neiting, Chongyang, Gongsun. Deficiency of *Yin*: Shangxing, Chize, Hegu, Taixi, Feiyang.

114. Swelling and Sore Throat

Prescription: wind-fire: Hegu, Shaoshang, Fengchi, Taiyuan, Pianli. Stagnated heat in the stomach and lung: Hegu, Shaoshang, Neiting. Deficiency of *Yin*: Hegu, Yuji, Taixi, Feiyang.

115. Stenocardia

Prescription: Neiguan, Ximen, Tiantu, Danzhong, Xinshu, Jueyinshu. Select 2-3 points every time, twirling the needle for several minutes, retaining needle for about 15-20 minutes.

116. Acute Cholecystitis, Cholelithiasis

Prescription: Yanglingquan, Zhongwan, Danshu.
Point Modification—vomiting: add Neiguan, Zusanli. Hypochondriac pain: add Riyue, Taichong.

117. Choleverminosis

Prescription: Yingxiang, Renzhong, Yanglingquan, Dannang (1-2 *cun* below Yang-lingquan).
Point Modification—vomiting: add Neiguan, Zusanli. For ascaris: Sifeng, Daheng.

图书在版编目(CIP)数据

针灸穴位层次解剖图谱:英文/高华龄编著 .—北京:外文出版社,1999
ISBN 7 - 119 - 01753 - 5

Ⅰ.针… Ⅱ.高… Ⅲ.穴位－解剖－图谱－英文 Ⅳ.R224.4－64

中国版本图书馆 CIP 数据核字 (95) 第 04113 号

责任编辑　刘文渊
封面设计　唐　宇
绘　　图　盛新农　蔡　荣　李士仅　唐　宇

外文出版社网址:
　　http://www.flp.com.cn
外文出版社电子信箱:
　　info@flp.com.cn
　　sales@flp.com.cn

针灸穴位层次解剖图谱
高华龄　编著
＊
ⓒ外文出版社
外文出版社出版
(中国北京百万庄大街 24 号)
邮政编码 100037
外文印刷厂印刷
中国国际图书贸易总公司发行
(中国北京车公庄西路 35 号)
北京邮政信箱第 399 号　邮政编码 100044
1999 年(16 开)第 1 版
(英)
ISBN 7 - 119 - 01753 - 5/R·122(外)
14000(精)
14 - E - 3012S